SLIM AND HEALTHY
WITHOUT DIETING

*The Weight Loss Solution for
Women over 40*

Dr. Khandee Ahnaimugan

Takagi Press

ISBN: 9781468006995

Published by Takagi Press
1st Printing January 2012
2nd Printing October 2015
ISBN: 1468006991

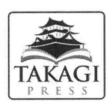

To my parents and my wife

Also by Dr Khandee Ahnaimugan:

Losing Weight After 40:
Change Your Life Without Dieting or Deprivation

For more help on your weight loss journey
Visit: www.doctorkweightloss.com

CONTENTS

INTRODUCTION

A woman walks up to a river. Although the water is raging, she sees a group of people trying to cross. They are wading through the torrents of water with their possessions held over their heads. It looks risky and dangerous.

As the woman watches, she sees one of the people lose their footing and fall over, getting swept away.

She is horrified and calls out to them to stop. One of the people, already knee deep in water, turns to her and says, "But we want to cross the river and this is the only way to go."

The woman looks further up the river. She can see something shining in the distance. She runs further upstream, and as she rounds the bend of the river she sees a gleaming new bridge.

She calls out to the people wading through the water, "I've found a bridge!" But they ignore her. They are too busy trying to cross the river.

If we think of trying to lose weight as crossing a river, then a diet is similar to wading through the raging torrents with your belongings held over your head. It's not easy and it's probably not going to end happily.

But most people persist in trying to cross the river this way because they are unaware of a better alternative. Like a shiny new bridge further upstream, there is a better, easier, safer way to lose weight.

In my weight loss practice my focus is exclusively on women over 40. I feel that the challenges they face in trying to achieve the benefits of weight loss are unique. Their needs are different from, say, a 25-year-old woman or a 45-year-old man.

And that shouldn't surprise us. Just like you wouldn't wear someone else's shoes and expect them to fit, you wouldn't expect a solution to someone else's weight problems to be exactly the same as for you.

Does this describe you?
If you're a woman over 40, does any of the following sound familiar?

- A slow increase in weight over a few years that you feel powerless to stop
- Slowing metabolism (you may feel like the amount you eat hasn't changed that much, but you're still gaining weight)
- Changing body shape with menopause

- Increasing exercise doesn't seem to make a difference
- A fear that you may never be slim again

The first thing to realise is that these experiences are common. Many women over 40 experience these changes and fears. And of course they can be both worrying and frustrating.

Many women I have seen tell me that they were at the end of their tether with their weight. It was slowly accumulating and they felt powerless. They had lost control of their own bodies.

There is a solution to this, but it is not to be found by following the crowd. Most people turn to diets as their solution. And dieting is not the way to lose weight, especially given the needs of women over 40.

My clients tell me that they:

1. Want a long-term solution to their weight loss. More so than any other group, women who are over 40 have tried many other weight loss approaches. They are sick of dieting. They want to lose weight once and for all.
2. Are less taken in by quick fixes and crash diets. In their twenties and thirties they were able to get quick (short-term) results from crash diets,

but after 40 these diets no longer work. As a result, women over 40 have a more realistic and mature approach to weight loss.

3. Are busy. They are often juggling busy jobs, families and active social lives. They don't have time to fit complicated diets into their lifestyle. Diets that require overhauls of their fridges and menus are too difficult to implement.

4. Want a solution that doesn't require starvation. They don't want to suffer to lose weight. They want to do things gently and sensibly.

5. Want to be able to enjoy life. Being on a "diet" is no fun. They want to be able to eat out and travel and enjoy themselves rather than be miserable on an extreme deprivation diet.

If you look at this list, you will realise that there is actually nothing unreasonable in any of these requirements. They are, in fact, sensible criteria. A long-term approach makes perfect sense.

Many of my clients, by the time they see me, have "diet fatigue". They are exhausted from having been on so many diets. Why would you want to keep putting yourself through that? Isn't it much better to have a solution to your weight that is permanent?

And of course, the greatest chance of a weight loss programme working is if it fits seamlessly into your life. If it requires a lot of extra work then you'll likely ditch the programme overboard as soon as you get busy or something disrupts your regular schedule.

How many people's diets have been thrown off course when they got busy at work or went on holiday?

The reason this happens is because the weight loss programme is too rigid and too time consuming. It relies too heavily on the person being able to devote large amounts of time and planning to make it work.

Similarly, the less enjoyable a diet is, the less likely you will continue with it. The only way a weight loss programme can work is if you stick with it. And this means it needs to be flexible enough to handle all the situations that come your way.

In this book, I'm going to show you how you can:

- Lose weight without dieting
- Lose weight while eating out, travelling and enjoying life

- Fit in a weight loss programme without having to overhaul your life
- Lose weight for the long term and avoid yo-yo dieting

1

WHY DIETS FAIL: THE KEY TO LASTING WEIGHT LOSS

A client once said to me in our very first session, "Saying you can help me lose weight without dieting is a pretty big claim!"

As you'll see in this chapter, it's not a big claim at all.

I'm going to show you why going on a diet is the completely wrong way to go about weight loss, and how the shortcoming of diets contains within it the seed for the true secret to long-term weight loss.

To begin with, let's be clear on what a diet is. When I talk about a diet I'm referring to a

1. Temporary
2. Severe restriction of food
3. In order to lose weight

You know what I'm referring to: when you stop eating what you normally eat and switch to eating much, much less for a short period of time, hoping that doing so will lead to weight loss.

So what is wrong with diets?

The fundamental flaw of a diet is that it's focused on the short term. As you see in the definition of a diet, it's a temporary restriction of food. Think about how most people talk about diets:

— *"My diet starts tomorrow."*
— *"I am going to slim down for my wedding."*
— *"I need to shed some pounds before I go on holiday."*

I think we can all agree that eating is an activity that most of us intend to do for the rest of our life.

If you are doing something for the rest of your life, it stands to reason that a short-term fix is not a long-term solution.

Just like you wouldn't brush your teeth once and think that your teeth were healthy for life, a short-term diet is not the way that you manage your weight for the rest of your life.

As an example, meet Helen.

Helen is fifty years old and is about two stone (28 pounds or 13 kilograms) above her ideal weight. Helen's weight has increased slowly over the last two years.

If you looked at her day-to-day activities you would see that certain parts of her lifestyle contribute to her gaining weight. In her example these include eating large portions at mealtimes, eating lots of high-calorie foods and not getting enough physical activity.

So Helen decides to go on a diet. As part of this diet, she has to drastically reduce the amount of food she eats and stop eating all the "bad" foods she normally enjoys. Obviously, this isn't easy, but Helen reasons that the short-term pain will be worth it, once she sees the results.

Let's say Helen is able to stick with the diet, despite its difficulties, and manages to lose weight. That in itself is an achievement, but once she's lost the weight, then what?

Once she's lost the weight, then what?

The diet is too strict to stick with for the rest of her life. But, if Helen stops the diet and goes back to doing the things she used to do, then she'll gain back the weight.

The elements of her lifestyle that made her over-weight (the large portions, the high-calorie foods, and the low physical activity) are all still there. They were temporarily put on hold for the diet, but once the diet is over, they're back.

This is a crucial point. If your lifestyle remains the same, then any time you aren't dieting, you're gaining back weight.

And that's the major shortcoming of using diets to lose weight. Diets are designed to get you to lose weight, but there is no thought to what happens after you've finished the diet.

Most diets that people go on are too unpleasant to continue indefinitely. They are, in fact, made intention-ally extreme in order to deliver rapid weight loss that people want. But this rapid weight loss, even if it comes, isn't sustainable.

And if you don't continue with the new eating plan and instead return to your pre-diet lifestyle, then you'll be doing the things that you did that got you overweight in the first place and so you'll gain the weight back.

In Helen's case, because she can't stick with the diet (it's too harsh), she must return to her old way of life, which means she'll gain back the weight she previously lost. Until she finds another diet.

In other words, she's trapped in a cycle of losing weight then gaining it back: yo-yo dieting.

The fact is, if your normal lifestyle is one that leads you to gain weight, then any diet will be like placing a sticking plaster on a festering sore.

You cannot expect to "cure" yourself of a weight-increasing lifestyle with a few weeks or months on a short-term diet.

The fact is: it's not hard to lose weight; it's just really hard to lose weight *on a diet*.

Does cutting back what I eat down to starvation levels help me lose weight quickly?
Eating more makes you gain weight, and eating less makes you lose weight. But as logical as it sounds, eating almost nothing does *not* make you lose weight faster.

This is because of the mechanisms we evolved to cope with periods of scarce food.

We can think of these mechanisms much like we think of a thermostat attached to a heater. When a room has a heater attached to a thermostat, as the temperature gets colder, the thermostat makes the heater turn on, to bring the temperature back up.

When the heater is on and the room gets too warm, then the thermostat kicks in again and the heater stops.

Our body weight is regulated in much the same way. The body tends towards homeostasis, meaning it tries to keep things in balance.

When you embark on a deprivation diet, the body reacts in much the same way as it would if you were in a famine. It goes into starvation mode (like a thermostat kicking in).

Now, instead of your body helping you, it starts to fight you.

It resists all attempts to lose weight. It holds on to fat (energy stores). You become preoccupied with food. Your desire for food broadens from a normal focus to dreaming of the most fat-drenched, sugar-laden food.

Of course, this all makes sense when you are in the middle of a famine, but:

> *The problem is that your body can't tell the difference between a famine and a fad diet.*

Fad diets put the body into starvation mode.

Starving yourself now and worrying about how to maintain it later

I've heard some people who've gone on really tough diets say that they knew that they wouldn't be able to maintain the brutal regime for the long-term, but they were only using it as a means of *losing* weight.

Once they got to their desired weight, they would "switch" to healthy ways of maintaining their weight.

But this reminds me of the story of the politician who lies, bribes and uses dirty tricks against his opponents in order to win an election thinking that he'll be able to "switch" to being high minded and honest after the election.

Of course, the idea of someone being dishonest to get into power and then suddenly being honest after that is laughable. You just can't do it. The manner in which you get somewhere affects how you go on.

And the same applies to weight loss. If you starve yourself to lose weight, it will be very hard to suddenly switch to a healthier, sustainable lifestyle once you get to your goal.

Isn't the key to weight loss just willpower?

No discussion about losing weight is complete without mentioning willpower.

The willpower myth is a very widespread and persistent one. I have met many people who believe that willpower is the missing ingredient in their weight loss. And more often than not, they believe that they lack the "willpower gene", and that's why they're overweight.

If you believe that a lack of willpower is what is standing between you and weight loss, I have some very good news for you: the fact is, willpower is not the key to weight loss.

Using willpower for weight loss implies that you're resisting doing things that you want to do because you know you "shouldn't". People can use this kind of discipline for a short time, but this strategy is not sustainable over the long term.

The reason is that the urge to eat is so powerful. Stopping yourself from eating something tempting goes against your deepest inner programming. When our ancestors saw food they had to eat it, because they didn't know when the next meal would be.

So you can use self-discipline to resist this urge to eat, but the evidence is that willpower is a limited resource.[1]

Willpower requires energy, and when you're using willpower for one thing, it limits your ability to resist something else[2] (for example, window shopping for things you can't afford – in other words, depleting your willpower – makes it hard to resist tempting food that is offered later).

Similarly, when under stress, your self-control is diminished. You might be able to resist that chocolate cake when things are going well in your life, but it is much more difficult after a bad day at work, as we all know.

Using willpower to stick to a diet is okay for a few weeks, but the idea of remaining self-disciplined about never eating chocolate or treats for the rest of your life isn't realistic.

So if willpower isn't the key, what is the real answer to weight loss? The answer is in the next chapter.

Chapter 1 Summary

1. Diets are a short term fix. You might be able to lose weight on a diet, *but then what?*
2. Whatever solution you choose to manage your weight should be for the long term.
3. Starving yourself to lose weight actually slows down your progress.
4. Willpower is *not* the key to weight loss.

2

HOW TO BE SLIM AND HEALTHY
WITHOUT DIETING

Most people know that diets don't work; usually from painful personal experience. And yet they still try them again and again, looking in vain for the perfect diet that will finally provide the answer.

Why?

You might say it's the triumph of hope over experience, but it's also because most people don't know of any other way.

But as we have seen in the previous chapter, the concept of dieting is flawed.

As long as your underlying lifestyle is one that causes weight gain, then you could go on "the best diet in the world", but as soon as you return to the old eating pattern, you will gain weight again.

In other words, you haven't discovered the best diet in the world; you've discovered the best yo-yo diet in the world.

But here we see the seed of our solution: your lifestyle.

What is your lifestyle?

It's your daily pattern of behaviours.

If there was a way to change your lifestyle, then you would be fixing the underlying problem.

Instead of slapping a diet on top of your existing lifestyle for a short time and hoping for the best, you would be dealing with the problem itself.

This would make it much more likely that you could accomplish long-term change: in other words, lasting weight loss.

But is there a way to change your underlying lifestyle?

Yes.

The answer involves making changes to your lifestyle to create lasting weight loss and then managing your weight for the rest of your life without resorting to diets or deprivation.

We can divide this weight loss solution into three parts:

1. Change your behaviour in a way that you are able to eat less without sacrificing your lifestyle.
2. Focus on changing your habits and thoughts to achieve long-term weight loss.
3. Take a gradual, sustainable approach.

1. **Eating less without sacrificing your lifestyle**

One of the things that distinguishes my weight loss programme from others is the principle that it is possible to eat what you want and still lose weight. This isn't a flashy promise designed to get attention, but actually the basis for the entire programme.

But how could it possibly work?

There exists a vast amount of research on different techniques that can help people lose weight. This research has been going on for many decades.

I collected information on all these different methods and came up with a database of behavioural modifications that satisfy three criteria:

1. They must be safe.
2. They must be effective in helping a person eat less.
3. They must allow the person to eat less while maintaining the same level of satisfaction from their eating.

This third point is crucial.

As you will see throughout this book, there are many, many ways that you can eat less in ways that leave you as satisfied (and sometimes more satisfied).

In fact, interwoven throughout this book are over 200 strategies that can allow you to eat less without feeling deprived.

Therefore, this programme is based on a set of behavioural modifications that allow people to eat what they want while still losing weight.

You're going to learn how to change your behaviour around eating so that you can eat less but still get the same level of satisfaction.

And if you eat less, you'll lose weight.

Time and again I've shown clients how this is possible and they've applied these changes to their lives with great success.

2. **Changing habits**

As I have discussed, diets are a short-term solution to weight gain. The real focus should be on changing your lifestyle. This is the key to a behavioural approach.

Another way of looking at the daily behaviours that make up your lifestyle is to think of them as habits.

Habits are actions that you repeat again and again in a similar situation.

For example, a habit may be that when you wake up in the morning you brush your teeth. With repetition, actions become automatic, so you don't even have to think about them; but they are still there.

With this in mind, have you noticed that when you try to lose weight it sometimes feels like you're fighting against yourself to make changes?

This is because you're trying to change your life without changing your habits. These habits have come about from repeated actions over a long period of time.

Once habits are entrenched, it's harder to introduce new behaviours. The average diet attempts to enforce a totally different way of doing things on top of your pre-existing habits.

This is why sticking to the latest fad diet is such hard going and why it feels so good to come off it.

What this means is that the superior approach is to focus on changing your existing habits.

If you change your habits, you change your behaviours and hence your results.

This programme is about applying those behaviours that allow you to eat what you want and still eat less in a way that you keep doing forever.

There are three parts to this process:

 – We need to establish the right foundations for making the change. To change a habit and behaviour requires a concerted effort and considerable energy. You need to feel that the action is worth the effort. This will be covered in Chapter 3: Laying the Foundations

– The new habit must be easy to apply and easy to become entrenched. The bulk of this book is dedicated to showing you behavioural modifications that are easy to apply to your life.

– You need to pay attention to how to maintain the habit for the rest of your life. This will be covered in Chapter 16: Staying Slim.

By focusing on these methods, you can change your habits and therefore your lifestyle: this is the ticket to long-term change and the escape from yo-yo dieting.

3. **Taking a gradual approach**

It is part of our nature to seek out the quick fix. And many people spend their lives searching for the perfect diet that will deliver them instantaneous weight loss with minimal effort. Of course, it doesn't exist.

In fact, the desire for urgent weight loss is actually the enemy of losing weight. The faster you want to lose weight, the more likely you'll make short-term changes instead of what is necessary for lifelong transformation.

In my weight loss clinic, if a woman comes to me and says, "I need to lose two stone (28 pounds) of weight in one month for my daughter's wedding", I tell her that I cannot work with her.

Someone who needs to lose so much so soon will not make the right decisions when losing weight.

She will be less interested in modifying habits and more interested in doing whatever she can to starve herself down to her desired weight by the deadline.

And who can blame her? But it's not the way I work.

I help women reach their desired weight in the safest, healthiest way possible and I do it in a way that allows them to maintain the weight loss for the long term.

A key part of this is the principle of small, gradual changes. Rather than asking you to make drastic cuts in what you eat, we make small changes each week.

Over time, we add more and more changes that add up to create big changes overall.

I also use the principle of successive approximation.

This means that we aren't aiming to completely change behaviour overnight. We're aiming to gradually refine your approach, so that you develop new ways of doing things.

Built into this is the fact that you'll probably make mistakes (as you refine your approach); there is no concept of failure.

Instead, we focus on taking steps that get us closer and closer to the goal.

So, instead of having short-lived failures from trying too much too soon, you get a track record of success behind you that you can build on.

The beauty of the gradual approach is that focusing on small changes over time is a much gentler way of doing things.

You never feel like you're starving. In some cases the changes feel so small that some clients say they feel like they aren't doing enough. But they are.

The key lesson is that a weight loss approach only works if you stick to it. And you maximise your chances of sticking to it by making it as easy as possible. This principle underlies everything I'll talk about in the rest of this book.

The details

This book explores this unique approach in depth.

You'll learn the behaviours that you need to develop to manage your weight successfully.

And you'll learn practical strategies and tools to make the changes that I use every day with my individual clients.

What's more, throughout this process I will be emphasising two important points that makes this weight loss programme quite different to others:

1. You will learn how to enjoy life while still managing your weight.
2. You will learn how to manage your weight for the long term. No more yo-yo dieting.

Chapter 2 Summary

1. If you want to lose weight for the long term, you need to change your underlying habits.
2. It's possible to eat less without sacrificing enjoyment.
3. Making small, gradual changes is the easiest way to lose weight and keep it off.

3

LAYING THE FOUNDATIONS: THE CAN'T-FAIL WAY TO LOSE WEIGHT

Motivation is a very important part of losing weight. But it's often misunderstood.

It's true of any attempt at behaviour change that you can't get someone to do something unless they really want to. So the question to ask yourself is: do you really want to lose weight?

This might seem like a ridiculous question. But the fact is, many people will say that they want to lose weight, but when you lay out a plan that they have to commit to, suddenly they're too busy, they don't have the time, or they think of some other excuse to avoid getting started.

What we're talking about here is motivation. And motivation is essential, because if you aren't strongly motivated to lose weight, you'll very likely give up at the first sign of a setback.

So what drives motivation?

In a study based on the National Weight Control Registry[1] (which is a database of people who have lost and kept off weight), 83 per cent had a triggering event as the driver behind their weight loss.

This included a medical trigger (for example, back pain, fatigue, sore joints), an emotional trigger (for example, "my husband left me") or a lifestyle trigger (for example, "I want to look good for my daughter's wedding").

If you haven't had a triggering event, you need to look for one! This means working out your reasons for needing to lose weight. And the fact is, if you're overweight, you really shouldn't need to look too hard to find reasons to lose weight.

Here are some positive reasons for wanting to lose weight. These are things that would happen if you managed to lose weight:

– Feeling more confident
– Feeling healthier

- Feeling more attractive
- Fitting into stylish new clothes
- Feeling more in control

Here are some reasons for losing weight that involve things that would happen if you *didn't* lose weight:

- Health problems like diabetes, heart disease, stroke, back pain, knee problems
- Feeling out of control
- Moving up a dress size
- Feeling self-conscious
- Lowered confidence
- Feeling less attractive

I include the negative reasons here because often people delude themselves into thinking that the choice they're faced with is either:

1. Lose weight.
2. Do nothing.

In this case, it would be very tempting to choose option number two, since it seems much easier. But the real choice is actually either:

1. Lose weight.
2. Suffer the consequences of being overweight and possibly also have your weight increase further.

A client once said to me her greatest fear was not that she was overweight, but that she'd had no control over her weight getting to where it was, and so there was nothing to stop it continuing to rise.

Look over those reasons for losing weight and add your own. Think how each applies to your life. Each of these reasons, when related to your life, will either be a "should" or a "must" reason.

When you say you *should* lose weight, there is a lack of urgency or conviction behind the words.

For example: "My clothes are getting tighter, so I should try to lose weight."

Compare this to: "My jeans feel so tight. I must do something about my weight."

The *must* reason has much more conviction and personal resonance. The stronger the must, the more you are driven to act and to persist.

If you genuinely review your reasons for losing weight, it's difficult to come to any other conclusion than that it would be desirable for you to lose weight.

Very few people could read that list and decide they had nothing to gain by taking action.

So what stops us? Well, the second aspect of motivation after the reasons why you want to lose weight, is your belief in your ability to do something about it. This comes down to two questions:

–   Do you believe that the particular weight loss method you are considering works?
–   Do you believe that you personally can lose weight using this method?

Most people I talk to are very doubtful about any methods of weight loss and certainly have grave doubts about their own ability to lose weight.

This isn't surprising.

There is a general feeling that losing weight is difficult and that most people fail. The preponderance of fad diets promising big results and not delivering doesn't help.

Previous disappointments hang heavily over many people I meet and undermine their belief in their ability to lose weight.

This is where a behavioural approach to weight loss is very powerful.

With standard diets, you either stick to them or you don't. If you stick to them, you're succeeding.

If you don't stick to them, you've failed.

With a behavioural approach, there's no way of failing.

Each change is attempted and if it doesn't work, it's either refined or discarded and a new strategy is used.

You're seeing what works and what doesn't. There isn't the pressure of sticking to something flawlessly (for more on this, see Chapter 5: Progress Not Perfection).

Secondly, a lack of previous success should not put you off.

With the people on the National Weight Control Registry[2] (mentioned earlier), 91 per cent described previous failed attempts prior to succeeding.

In general, with any kind of behaviour change, most people aren't successful on their first attempt. Failed attempts should be looked at as steps closer to the goal, not steps further away.

Thirdly, don't interpret doubts as a lack of motivation.

Because so many people these days have tried "dieting", we all have a track record of a weight loss attempts that failed. This doesn't mean anything.

In fact, I can't think of a single client I have had who didn't have doubts. Doubts are normal.

You must separate out your desire to lose weight (which may be strong) from your bad experiences in the past (which aren't relevant to your current plan to lose weight).

This can be difficult but it's essential. Your doubts must not get in the way of you taking action.

Once people take action and start to see results they're filled with greater confidence. This makes it easier to continue.

But I notice with some of my clients that even as they lose weight they may still have doubts. This is important to acknowledge, because it shows that having doubts isn't a barrier to weight loss.

Goal setting
Setting a motivating and achievable goal is a crucial part of the weight loss process. If you don't know where you want to go, how will you know when you get there?

To set a realistic goal, we need to see where you are right now. I use two measurements: the BMI and the waist circumference.

BMI
You calculate BMI by dividing your weight in kilograms by your height in metres squared. Once you've worked out your BMI, then you need to look at what the different results mean. Here's a quick guide:

BMI categories:

> Underweight = <18.5
> Normal weight = 18.5–24.9
> Overweight = 25–29.9
> Obese = BMI of 30 or greater

BMI is a useful measure but it does have its limitations.

It may overestimate body fat in athletes and others who have a muscular build. It doesn't take into account body shape, or differences between ethnic groups.

And it may also underestimate body fat in older persons and others who have lost muscle. But having said that, in most people BMI gives a decent idea of whether a person is overweight or not.

Waist circumference
The other important measurement is the waist circumference, which is directly related to how much fat you have in your abdomen.

Having fat on your abdomen is a very accurate marker of your risk of developing certain conditions like type 2 diabetes and heart disease.

This is what is often referred to as the apple- and pear-shaped bodies.

People who carry more weight in their middle ("apple shaped") are more at risk than people who carry it around their hips ("pear shaped").

Women are more likely to have pear-shaped bodies than men, but after menopause, this changes.

This is why many of my clients notice after menopause that they gain weight around their abdomen. They also report having trouble fitting into their jeans, because of the movement of weight from their hips to their stomachs.

To measure waist circumference, the tape measure should be roughly around the level of the belly button. The tape measure needs to be placed midway between the lower rib and the hip bone.

You need to fully breathe out when you take the measurement and there should be no tension in your abdomen.

The measurement should be read from the side, not the front.

- For women, a "not overweight" reading is less than 80cm. Between 80 and 88 centimetres is overweight and above 88 centimetres is obese.
- For men, a "not overweight" reading is less than 94cm. Between 94 and 102 centimetres is overweight. And above 102 centimetres is obese.

To weigh or not to weigh
In the past, when working with clients I used to try to de-emphasise the importance of weight. This was because I felt that it could be dangerous to focus too

much on scales. Measuring weight can be misleading. In short-term (fad) diets a big initial drop is more often related to losing water than losing fat.

The biggest reason that I didn't want my clients weighing themselves regularly was that I was concerned that focusing on weight readings made some people go through roller-coasters of emotion depending on what the scales showed.

The worst case is if someone reacts to a higher-than-expected weight measurement with either a drastic restriction of intake (which I don't support) or giving up altogether (which I also don't support).

Conversely, when the scales are showing a drop, some people get complacent or even reward themselves by eating more food.

I've since changed my stance on clients weighing themselves during the programme. Most people need to have some sense of achievement week-to-week and a falling weight often helps with this. But weighing always needs to be kept in context, because one reading means nothing on its own.

Setting the goal
Once you've worked out your BMI and waist circumference, it's time to set a goal.

It's okay to have an *eventual* target weight in mind, but what I do with my clients is set an *initial* goal.

If you need to lose four stone (56 pounds), that's a large goal and can seem very daunting. Even really good progress may not feel adequate when you compare it to a large goal.

That's why, with most of my clients the initial goal is one stone (fourteen pounds or 6.3 kilograms). This is really the ideal target, since for most people losing one stone will make a real difference in their lives and yet it is an achievable goal that is not too overwhelming.

Once you get to one stone, you can set a new goal.

But I do want to say a few words about setting the final goal for how much weight you want to lose.

We live in a world where the relentless message drummed into us is that slimmer is better. While there is benefit to reducing weight for health reasons, for many people the images they see on TV and magazines set up completely unrealistic expectations of the goals that they want to achieve.

I know people who genuinely believe that a woman can only be healthy when she resembles a supermodel (even though many models may have BMIs that fall into the underweight category) and that a man can only be healthy when he has washboard abs.

This is a recipe for unhappiness.

The fact is, for many of us, the practical, realistic weight that we can achieve will be well short of catwalk standards.

Achieving a weight that could land us on magazine covers would require deprivation of food on a level that would guarantee nothing but misery.

For others our basic builds simply make that kind of body unattainable.

What we need to look at is whether our weight goals are sabotaging our happiness.

Is aiming for the fashion magazine dream weight helping you to be healthy and happy?

Or would it be better to aim for a healthy, realistic weight that you can achieve and maintain?

If you can do this, you can make your weight loss journey much easier and more rewarding. And remember, there are health benefits from losing even 5 per cent of your weight.[3]

Chapter 3 Summary

1. Look at your reasons for losing weight.
2. Remember that previous failures to lose weight don't mean anything. You can still succeed.

3. A behavioural approach isn't pass/fail. You learn from mistakes and continue to modify your behaviour. You can't fail at this approach, so relax.
4. Work out a good initial goal. Make it achievable and motivating. One stone (14 pounds or 6.3 kilograms) is often a good start.
5. Be realistic about your eventual goal. Don't sacrifice happiness by chasing an unrealistic weight.

4

THE MAGIC MARGIN: HOW YOU CAN EAT LESS AND NOT FEEL HUNGRY

I magine being able to eat like a gourmet and still lose weight. Imagine being one of those people who seems to eat what they want and still stays slim.

These are alluring promises, and perhaps so alluring that, on the face of it, they sound like celebrity fad diet claims. In other words: too good to be true.

And when we hear something that sounds too good to be true, a part of us gets excited, but we're also scared of having our hopes dashed in case it's just a bold claim with no grounding in reality.

But the fact is, you *can* eat what you want and still lose weight. You can eat out, travel, enjoy life and still be slim. How? By using the magic margin.

What's the magic margin? It's the unnecessary parts of your eating that you can eliminate to lose weight.

The magic margin is the unnecessary parts of your eating that you can eliminate to lose weight

Let's be clear: if you want to lose weight, you have to reduce how much you eat; that much is certain.

But instead of the standard "scorched earth" approach of most diets, where you're left eating almost nothing, the magic margin allows you to make transformative changes to the amount you eat without compromising your lifestyle.

Clients of mine have managed to reduce the calories they take in, while still enjoying a diet that's remarkably similar to the one they had before they started losing weight.

When you think about that, it's quite amazing.

Most people are put off from trying to lose weight because they fear the deprivation of a standard diet, and yet, by using the magic margin, it's possible to eat much the same diet and still lose weight.

Not just that, but it's possible to do this without affecting your enjoyment and way of life.

I understand that this might seem paradoxical, so let me explain further.

The best way to understand this is to look at the main reasons why we eat food.

The most obvious reason is that we eat food because we need nutrients for energy and growth. But it's also fair to say that, for most of us, food also serves other legitimate needs.[1] After all, eating is enjoyable. We eat because it's fun.

If you look at most diets, this distinction, that food also serves enjoyment needs, is missing.

Most diets reduce food down to necessity value only as a means of getting to the goal as fast as possible.

No thought is given to how a person can live the rest of their life on such a regime.

Of course, with most diets, there is no thought about long-term considerations because it's all about the short term.

I have had clients telling me about previous attempts to lose weight, where they had to give up on particularly brutal deprivation diets because they felt like torture.

But of course, the harder these diets are, the less likely you are to stick to them.

In other words the easier you can make your weight loss programme, the better.

You don't have to suffer to lose weight.

If we accept that we consume food because we have nutritional needs but also for enjoyment, not only do we have a more realistic view of food, but we can use this to change our eating for the better.

Are there instances when the food we eat neither gives us nutrients nor provides us with satisfaction? The answer is yes.

Here's an example from a situation where you think you're satisfying your hunger but actually you're not.

You've just had a nice meal at a restaurant and the waiter gives you the dessert menu. You really feel the craving for something sweet so you order a sorbet.

When the sorbet arrives, you take a bite. It's very tasty. You made a great choice.

But after the third bite, it becomes less enjoyable.

By the time you reach the last bite, you're just eating it because you want to finish what's on your plate.

In this instance, the first few bites were enjoyable, but once you'd satisfied your craving, the rest of the dessert was not.

It didn't contribute any real nutritional value, and it wasn't particularly enjoyable.

If you had stopped eating after a few mouthfuls you would have saved maybe 200 to 300 calories.

In which case, you haven't lost any nutrition (it's sorbet, after all), you haven't lost any enjoyment and you've lost certain calories that you would have had to work off or lose in the future.

Remember, a calorie saved is a calorie lost.

In this example, the extra eating was food that didn't contribute any extra enjoyment to your life. But by continuing to eat it, you needlessly put calories into your body, therefore increasing your weight.

This range of eating, where you get neither enjoyment nor nutrition, is what I call the magic margin.

Why?

Because it's in this margin of your eating that you can cut out food in a way that your body doesn't miss out on nutrients and you don't miss out on enjoyment.

You get a disproportionately powerful effect just from making some small changes.

This book is filled with insights into how you can apply the magic margin to your life.

There are over 200 areas in which you may be eating needlessly and contributing to your weight without any increase in enjoyment. If you eliminate this magic margin, you lose weight but not enjoyment.

Here are just a few examples of where you can find the magic margin in your life:

1. Eating while watching the TV. Often you're eating snacks that aren't healthy, and while in a trance-like state while watching the box you don't even take the time or awareness to really enjoy what you're eating. These are empty, unnecessary calories.
2. Eating out of habit; for example, always having second servings.
3. Eating to time; for example, always eating lunch at twelve p.m. even if you're not hungry.
4. Unnecessary variety; for example, at a buffet, always taking food from every dish, even though you don't enjoy most of them.

The key, then, is to stick to foods that are healthy and foods that you love to eat (and of course, sometimes a particular food can be both).

And when I say love, I mean *adore*.

Not "mediocre" food.

Not "might as well because it's here" food.

But really mouth-watering foods.

You must become a hedonist. Only the best will do. Savour the taste of food that is enjoyable, including textures, smells and flavours.

Take your time, like a connoisseur appreciating a fine wine.

Dr. Rick Kausman, a GP in Melbourne, Australia, who does a lot of work with overweight and obese patients, tells his patients to ask themselves: "I can have it if I want it, but do I really feel like it?"[2] I have modified this slightly to:

> *"I can have it if I want to, but do I really need it right now?"*

The "I can have this if I want to" is important, because it emphasises that you're not depriving yourself.

The "do I really need it right now" is about prioritising your true needs for food as the primary reason you should consider before anything else.

"I can have it if I want to, but do I really need it right now?" is a good question to ask before you eat anything.

To paraphrase one of my clients: *"If I'm going to take in calories, I don't want to waste it on things I don't enjoy."*

Now you might think that limiting yourself to this kind of diet means that you would just be eating broccoli (healthy) and chocolate (tasty) all day long.

But the lesson here is not to change your usual diet completely, but to look at what you normally eat and eliminate those foods that fall in the magic margin.

The magic margin is how you can make weight loss a long-term process.

As I've said, unpleasantness in a weight loss programme must be avoided if you want to be at a healthy weight for the long term.

Look at your current diet. If you explore it in much the same way I do with my clients, you'll see many areas where you could make changes. The rest of this book will show you where to look and, most importantly, how to make these changes.

The beauty of the magic margin is that by taking away food from your diet you actually make things better. You feel better, less full or bloated, and are ready to enjoy food better and relish it more. As I like to say about food: *"If it's not healthy or heavenly then it's a hazard."*

This approach explains how my clients are able to lose weight, even though their diets don't look that much different from the average person's.

This is how you can eat less and still enjoy life to the maximum without giving up enjoyment.

Chapter 4 Summary

1. There is a portion of your eating that neither provides you with health benefits nor gives you enjoyment. This is the magic margin.
2. If you eliminate the magic margin, you can remove a significant amount of calories from your diet without noticing any effect on your enjoyment or health.

5

PROGRESS, NOT PERFECTION: THERE'S NO SUCH THING AS A BAD DAY

Have you ever tried to lose weight and thought things were going okay until one bad day knocked you off course? I hear this story a lot. Here's an example that may sound familiar:

Alison was on a "diet" and she was following the directions to the letter. She spent time each day planning what to eat since she could only eat food that was approved by the diet.

This also meant having a special shopping list and declining dinner invites from friends, in case they served her food that was off the diet.

She figured that this short-term denial would pay off in the long term.

Then the family went on holiday. Alison managed to limit herself to approved foods for the first day but eventually her resolve broke and she ended up "cheating" on her diet.

She was so angry with herself. She felt that her lack of willpower had ruined her weight loss attempt and so she gave up.

This is a very common scenario. How many diets have been sunk by a "bad" day? How many people have cheated on their diet (especially while on holiday), leading to complete meltdown?

This kind of talk of bad days and cheating is so prevalent and so symptomatic of the diet culture. Even people who say they know that diets are no good still speak about their weight loss in those terms.

But is it realistic to want to lose weight without having a bad day? Is it realistic to change any kind of behaviour or develop any new habit without slipping up every now and then?

Imagine a child learning to ride a bike. We don't expect the child to be able to jump on a bike for the first time and start pedalling. And if the child falls off (which is highly likely) we don't tell them off and advise them to give up trying.

And yet so many women have a "bad" day on a diet and then decide to give up all together.

There are two elements to this that you need to change if you're going to lose weight successfully.

1. Eliminating the all-or-nothing approach to weight loss
2. Responding to "bad" days appropriately

The right approach

Most diets promote an all-or-nothing approach to weight loss. If you're following the diet perfectly, you're good. If you stray, you're bad.

But to stick to a rigid diet without straying is really the exception rather than the rule. The vast majority of people can't stick to a strict diet perfectly.

And yet, when someone strays, they act like they've done something terrible. They may feel guilt and disappointment, and might even think of giving up. This is exemplified by statements like: "Oh well, I stuffed things up, I might as well just have the entire tub of ice cream or bar of chocolate." This all-or-nothing approach sets people up for misery.

We need to accept that life is complicated, and that when you're trying to lose weight you're going to be put in situations where there's food that's not regarded as healthy.

And if you're on a diet where you can't have any of the foods you desire, then you're really setting yourself up for trouble. If your list of forbidden foods is extensive, then you'll eventually feel cravings for at least some of them, and it's hard to resist over time.

Not only do most diets have an all-or-nothing approach, but they expect people with less-than-perfect lifestyles to switch overnight to the perfect diet and then maintain it for the rest of their lives. How likely is that? Rather than trying to stick to a plan flawlessly, you're much better off trying to change your habits.

Rather than viewing weight loss as a matter of starting on a perfect diet immediately and sticking to it for the rest of your life, weight loss should instead be viewed as a process.

You're not trying to be perfect. You're just aiming for small changes that add up. It's through trial and error, seeing what works for you, that you get better and better.

How do you respond to "bad" days?
When you view weight loss as a process, you realise that bad days and even bad weeks are part of the process. And they're part of life. You don't ignore them or castigate yourself for letting them happen.

You work out what happened, and why it happened, and try to avoid it happening again.

You also proactively anticipate problems.

In the example at the beginning of the chapter, Alison could have been more realistic and acknowledged that being surrounded by temptation and relaxation was a danger point for her weight loss.

She could have anticipated challenges and made plans to deal with them. (Chapter 14: Having a Life explains how to deal with holidays and eating out, and Chapter 15: Chocolate Is Calling shows you how to deal with temptation.)

Here's an example of a client who dealt with a bad week in "the Dr. K way":

My client, Susan, had already lost about half a stone (about seven pounds or three kilograms) working with me. And then she had a particularly bad week. She ate much more than she usually would due to a combination of travel and business dinners.

Now, I'm pretty sure that if Susan hadn't had the benefit of someone to support her during this week (i.e. me), then this one bad week would have derailed her weight loss efforts, as it would with most people. Her progress in losing half a stone would have been thrown away. She would have thought, "What's the point? I can't stick to this", and then responded by over-eating even more.

Instead, Susan was able to maintain her perspective. She realised that one bad week wasn't the end of the world. She knew that she wanted to develop habits that lasted the rest of her life. And she accepted that in a regular busy life bad weeks will happen, and she needed to have better ways of dealing with them. The bad week was a spur to keep going, not to give up.

And happily, Susan continued to lose more weight after that, so far reaching two stone (28 pounds) of weight loss, and still going strong.

And so this is the difference between success and failure in weight loss. Failure means giving up after the first bad week. Success means keeping going.

Here's how to deal with a bad day in six easy steps:

1. Acknowledge that you strayed and ate more than you needed, and accept that it's not only inevitable but also that it doesn't need to derail your weight loss efforts.
2. Remind yourself that it's normal for eating to fluctuate from day to day.
3. Draw a line in the sand. Don't keep eating just because you had a small slip-up. It's very easy to say, "I can't believe I let myself down. I can't believe I ate that. I've really blown it. I might as well eat whatever I want for the rest of the day, and start dieting again tomorrow."

   But this sort of thinking makes the damage even worse. Stop eating and realise that every bite you have after the initial one is only contributing further calories that you'll either have to live with or try to burn off at a later date.
4. To stop yourself continuing to eat, do something totally different and try to leave the scene if possible.
5. Recommit to your goal. You have a goal in mind, be it feeling healthier, feeling more confident, or fitting into more stylish clothes, and you also have consequences you want to avoid such as heart attacks, strokes, poor self-esteem, and feeling tired all the time.

Remember the reasons that you want to lose weight, and continuously remind yourself of these.

6. Learn from the mistake. This is very important. I often have clients who don't like to tell me bad news (for example, they ate something they shouldn't have).

Firstly, there's no such thing as should or shouldn't.

And secondly, it's times when people stray from what they intended that we learn the most about the environment and factors that affect their eating.

When a client describes going off track, I want to know everything about it. Why did it happen? How did it happen? How can we avoid or eliminate the risk of this happening again?

So much valuable information can be gleaned from a "bad" day. Don't waste the opportunity.

And always remember: progress, not perfection.

"The scales aren't budging"

Have you ever felt like you were doing everything right, but when you checked the scales, there was no change? It can be frustrating and disillusioning, and enough for some people to throw in the towel.

A common reason for this reaction is the person not appreciating the natural pattern of weight loss. When my clients lose weight, one of the things that I almost always notice is that weight loss doesn't happen as a steady downward trend.

If someone is going to lose ten pounds over ten weeks, they don't lose one pound each week. Instead, more often than not there will be a few weeks with hardly any movement at all, and then a sudden drop. This is especially true of women.

Anyone familiar with weight loss will know of these times when weight loss slows or halts as *plateaus*, and they are very common. Why do they happen?

It comes down to the body and its inbuilt mechanisms for maintaining the status quo. The body always tries to maintain homeostasis. That is, if things change, it tries to compensate, to maintain things at the same level. This is the thermostat attached to the heater example I spoke about in Chapter 1. The body will fight back for any reduction in intake or increased burning of calories.[1,2]

So when you cut back what you're eating, the body can't tell if this is a famine or a diet. Its immediate response is to reduce metabolism to retain body stores of fat. But after a few weeks of reduced intake, when it appears that food isn't as scarce as initially thought, the body goes off high alert and relaxes a bit. The weight is allowed to drop.

This is why there is often a plateau period when trying to lose weight. You're doing all the right things, but the body isn't shedding fat until it can be certain that you're not starving to death because of lack of food in the environment.

This plateau can be a trap for young players. I have seen many clients start to feel doubtful about their weight loss efforts, because they don't see any evidence on the scales.

Some people can get so distraught over one bad scales reading that they give up on their weight loss efforts altogether.

But the scales aren't the place to be looking. Not only does weight loss happen in fits and starts, but your weight can fluctuate from day to day based on any number of factors including hydration, hormones and recent meals.

The thing to remember here is that the scales are nice indicators of progress (especially of trends of weight loss) but individual readings are meaningless. In

some contexts, even a few weeks of readings are unhelp-
ful because the weight sometimes takes a few weeks to
catch up with the changes that are being made.

What's more helpful is the food diary (See Chapter
Six for more on this). When good changes are evident
on the food diary, they become apparent a few weeks
later on the bathroom scales. There is a delay between
the good actions and the good results.

So don't let the scales fool you. And don't let plateaus and fluctuations throw you off. Maintain focus on
your food diary. When you've made the positive changes to your eating then there will inevitably be a delay
before you see the results.

This isn't the time to give up. You need to just maintain your patience.

As I say to my clients, you can't defy the laws of ther-
modynamics. If you're taking in less energy (assuming
your activity levels remain the same), you'll eventually
lose weight. No other outcome is possible in this uni-
verse we live in.

So what you really need is some patience as you
await the changes. The results will come. Just as people who are overweight can only gain weight by putting

food in their mouths, people who reduce what they eat will eventually lose weight.

The message here is that you need to focus on your eating, not the bathroom scales, because if you take care of what you're eating, the weight will take care of itself.

Chapter 5 Summary

1. Go easy on yourself. You don't need to stick perfectly to a diet to lose weight. This kind of all-or-nothing approach sets you up for failure and disappointment.
2. If you have a "bad" day, use it as a learning experience. Take steps to ensure that it doesn't happen again. And even if it does, keep trying. It's in your responses to mistakes that you improve.
3. Don't confuse plateaus or weight fluctuations with failure to progress. If you've cut down what you eat, you will lose weight. Be patient.

6

INDISPENSABLE ADVICE: IF YOU CAN ONLY DO ONE THING TO LOSE WEIGHT...DO THIS

I magine that both you and a friend decided to try to lose weight (since you're reading this book, that shouldn't be too hard to imagine).

Let's assume that you're both roughly the same weight and that you both limit your intake of food to lose weight (as opposed to increasing the amount of exercise you do).

If everything you did was identical, but you wrote down everything you ate and your friend didn't, what do you think would be the difference in weight loss? According to a study done in 2005[1], you might lose as much as two times more weight than your friend.

When people come to me asking for the simplest weight loss advice I can give (by the way, if someone asks for "simple" weight loss advice, you can almost guarantee that they aren't going to do anything about it), the first thing I tell them is to keep a food diary.

I once wrote a blog post where I said that if you only had 80 seconds a day to devote to losing weight, your best bet would be to spend that time recording what you had eaten.

And I truly believe this.

Why do food diaries work?
Keeping a food diary is a form of self-monitoring, which is one of the foundations of behavioural therapy. There are good reasons that self-monitoring is so important.

Firstly, self-monitoring increases your awareness of what you're doing.

For most of the women I see as clients, the number one reason that they've gained weight over a period of time is that they've stopped paying attention to what they're eating.

The weight creeps up on them like a ninja, a few pounds a year. Even three pounds a year can add up to fifteen pounds in five years and thirty pounds in ten years.

This gradual weight gain can be very confusing to some people who tell me: "I don't understand how I gained so much weight."

The fact is, even small differences in what you're eating can make a big difference over time. 100 extra calories a day (the amount in a can of cola) could add up to could add up to ten to fourteen pounds of extra weight in a year.

But, on the other hand, we can make use of the fact that small changes in the other direction can lead to **significant weight loss** over time too.

For others who aren't victims of the slow, gradual gain, the lack of awareness is due to some kind of stressful event, where their attention is diverted and they pay less attention to what they're eating. This can mean gaining large quantities of weight in a relatively short time.

In both cases, the key to regaining control of your eating is to regain awareness of what you're doing day by day. It's only with this awareness that you can be clear on what behaviours are causing you the most problems.

The more aware you are of what you're eating and how much you're eating, the less likely it is that weight gain sneaks up on you. This is what I aim for when working with clients. I want the awareness of what they're eating to become a habit. Awareness is the antidote to further unexpected weight gain.

So writing down what you eat (honestly) can immediately make you realise exactly how much you're eating every day.

Interestingly enough, simply having to write down what you eat can make you change your behaviour.[2] If you know you have to write down what you eat, you will immediately think twice about whether you should eat something or not and so adjust your food intake.[3]

As a client once said to me, "It's harder to have the fifth canapé if I know I have to write it down in my food diary and send it to you."

There are two interesting points to note with food diaries:

1. People tend to under-report what they're eating, especially when they're overweight. This has been shown time and time again in studies.[4,5]

In one study 81 per cent of people under-reported their daily eating. Women under-reported by approximately 428 calories, which was a massive 18 per cent of their daily intake.[6]

2. Food diaries must include weekends as well as weekdays, since most people tend to eat more on weekends than weekdays.[7]

The second advantage of the food diary is that it allows you to notice patterns in the way you eat.

Do you eat certain things at certain times of day? Do you eat when someone else is around? Do you eat more in certain places? This kind of information can be a goldmine.

When I'm working with a client and we discover a pattern to eating, it can literally transform the client's eating and therefore her weight.

How should I keep a food diary?
So how should you go about completing a food diary? There are different types of food diaries, varying in complexity. The simplest version is one where you just write down what you eat and when.

But food diaries can also include weighing how much you eat, calculating how many calories or points each item of food is, and detailing the circumstances of the meal.

I tend to go for the simplest alternative with my clients. I ask them to write down what they eat, and approximately when they eat it. This because the more complicated the food diary gets, the less likely it is that people will stick to it.

While I keep the recording part simple, when I sit down with my clients to review their food diary, that's when I ask a lot of questions. I want to know as much as I can about the circumstances in which they're eating. Here are some of the areas I cover:

- Why did you eat it?
- Where did you eat it?
- Were you hungry before you ate it?
- Were you satisfied after eating it?
- Were there any other factors that affected how much or what you ate (for example, habit, obligation, food availability)?
- If you could repeat the meal, what would you change?

These are the sorts of questions you need to ask yourself around what you eat. If you do this, you'll get a huge amount of information that you can then use to change your behaviour.

How long does it take to fill out a food diary? I've had varying reports: anything from eighty seconds to five minutes. Once you get into the habit, it can take less time.

When filling out the diary, try to do it as soon after the meal as possible. If you need to, keep a small notebook with you. Or maybe even enter it into your phone. The longer the time that elapses between eating and recording, the more that inaccuracies creep in. To illustrate this, try remembering what you had for lunch yesterday.

One of my clients once told me how she had written down what she had eaten but left the notebook at work. The next day, she had to send me her food diary, and so she completed the previous day's intake from memory.

When she eventually got to compare the two entries, she was shocked to see how different they were. And there had been only a day's difference between eating and recording. The biggest discrepancy almost always relates to snacks, which can easily slip the mind.

Getting someone else to look at your food diary can make things much more effective. This is a key aspect of what I do with my individual clients. Just knowing that someone else will have a look at the diary can alter your behaviour significantly.

I genuinely feel that a food diary is one of the most important parts of a weight loss programme. For a small investment of time each day, it has a powerful effect on your eventual results.

I make it compulsory for anyone working with me to fill in a food diary and if you are serious about getting the best results, you should make it a compulsory part of your weight loss programme too.

Chapter 6 Summary

1. A food diary is the simplest and best first step to losing weight.
2. Food diaries make you more aware of what you're eating and help you pick up patterns in your eating.
3. There are many types of food diary, and you should choose the type that suits you best.
4. Getting someone else to review your food diary is.

7

BALANCED INDULGENCE: HOW THAT WOMAN SEEMS TO EAT SO MUCH AND STILL STAYS SLIM

The friend we all love to hate

"*I have a friend called Sally whom I meet up with about once a month. We go out for dinner with our husbands. And every time we go out, she eats so much food. She has a starter, a main and dessert. And the most annoying thing is that she's really skinny!*"

Almost everyone knows someone like Sally. They seem to defy natural laws by being able to eat whatever they want and still stay slim.

And what would most people say is the reason for this? Genetics? Fast metabolism?

What would Sally herself say? Funnily enough, she would most likely say that she's just one of those lucky people who can eat what she wants and still not gain weight.

But the fact is, the most likely explanation for Sally's remarkable gift is not genetics, fast metabolism or luck, but simply that, overall, she eats less than others.

But how can that be? How does she eat less than others when her friend clearly sees Sally devouring a three-course meal in front of her? The difference is that Sally balances her indulgence.

What do I mean by balancing indulgence?

I mean compensating for a large, indulgent meal by reducing what you eat before and/or afterwards.

In other words, because Sally had such a large meal for dinner, she probably had a smaller-than-usual lunch. Or she may have reduced what she ate the next day.

By reducing what she eats in other meals, Sally is able to eat more when she goes out and therefore give her poor friend the illusion that she has a magic metabolism.

Contrast the balancing of intake that Sally practises with what an overweight person would do. No matter how big a meal is, an overweight person continues to eat the usual amount for the next meal. If they have an extra-large lunch, they still eat a regular dinner.

In fact let's be clear here: most people don't naturally compensate for larger meals.[1] And most people are overweight.

If an overweight person has a larger-than-usual lunch, they would still have a regular sized dinner. On the other hand, if Sally felt that she had eaten more than usual for lunch, she might have a lighter dinner.

The point is, she moderates what she eats by taking into account what she's already eaten and also what she's planning to eat later.

But please remember, most of this isn't conscious; it happens naturally. It's a habit. So in Sally's mind she feels like she can eat whatever she wants. This is because she forgets that she has subconsciously adjusted her eating.

And because it's all happening subconsciously, you will hear people like Sally say things like, "I feel so full after lunch; I don't feel like having much for dinner."

"But I know someone who genuinely does eat lots and is really slim"
Whenever I mention this concept of balanced indulgence, there's always someone who swears that they know a person who eats nothing but fast food and still doesn't gain weight.

Obviously, unless I meet this person I can't refute this. And unless one spends an entire week with them and has access to an accurate measure of what they've eaten, it's really hard to prove. But the main point to make is that these people they describe are never over 40.

And when I've met people who claim that they can eat what they want and not gain weight, it soon becomes apparent that they're subconsciously balancing what they eat during the day, or sometimes over a longer timeframe like several days.

A study done with adolescents eating fast food showed that overweight people tend to eat more, but as well as that, they don't compensate in other meals of the day. On the other hand, people of healthy weight tend to compensate. If they have fast food for lunch, they tend to reduce their intake afterwards.[2]

I remember giving a talk during which I asked the audience whether there was anyone there who felt like they could eat whatever they wanted and still not gain weight.

One woman put up her hand (and I should say that she got some dirty looks from others in the room).

I explained the idea of balanced indulgence and after the talk that same woman shared a story with me. She had always felt lucky that she was one of those people with a fast metabolism. But after hearing the talk, she realised that actually how she managed to eat what she wanted was by balancing her intake.

She recalled that earlier that week she had gone out for lunch with work colleagues and had an entire pizza. Her colleagues had watched with amazement as this very slim woman ate such a large lunch.

But she realised now that after that large meal she had subconsciously reduced what she had eaten *for the rest of the week.* She had not consciously thought about this, but looking back, it was clear to her.

How do you develop this ability?
It would appear that relying on a fast metabolism and lucky genes is unnecessary if you want to be one of those people who seem to eat what they want and not get fat.

What you need to do is increase your awareness of what you're eating and when you're having meals that are bigger than usual.

With my clients, this is achieved with the humble food diary. Looking at a food diary over a period of a week or so, you can start to notice patterns.

What do you do when you have a big meal? Do you adjust the meal after and the meal before accordingly? Or do you proceed as usual? Awareness of these patterns is the best way to realise whether you are balancing your intake or not.

I also like to get my clients to notice other people who, they think, are able to eat whatever they want. Don't just watch them for one meal; try to get an idea of what they're eating before and after. Are they limiting their intake at other times?

The advantage you have over the "naturally" thin
If someone balances their indulgence subconsciously, then they really aren't aware of what they're doing.

As I mentioned, Sally, the woman who eats large meals and yet remains a healthy weight, has no idea how she does it. And this makes her ill-prepared for any change in her circumstances.

As we get older our metabolism slows by 1 to 2 per cent per year. A woman in her fifties may need 400 fewer calories than when she was in her twenties.[3]

This explains why I can see people who were "slim all their life" complain of increasing weight after the age of 40.

Because they weren't actually aware of what they were doing (it just happened naturally), when their metabolism slowed down and the balance was tipped, they were suddenly not able to offset it.

Their weight drifted up, and they were powerless to stop it.

Now that you know the key to balanced indulgence, you'll be able to do what they couldn't.

What this means to you while losing weight
In practice, what this idea of balanced indulgence means for weight loss is that you're allowed to have a "bad" day when losing weight. One bad meal, day or week shouldn't derail what's going to be a lifetime of healthy, sensible eating.

Indeed, having a diet where you eat the same amount every day is unnatural and unlikely to be sustainable.

Some consistency helps, but most of my clients like variety in their meals.

And if you lead a normal, busy and socially active life, you'll be having very different meals and different experiences.

If you're not going to allow yourself to experience these while trying to lose weight, you'll despise your diet. You'll feel like it's a short-term venture. And you'll be craving the old life you had.

You might be able to maintain it for a short time, but by denying yourself your old pleasures, you're ensuring that you sabotage your progress.

If you're living a normal life, you'll have times when you're eating more than others. This doesn't mean you're being bad, but it does mean that you need to compensate. It does mean you need to practise balanced indulgence.

Fairness
I remember a client once complaining to me that it "didn't feel fair" that she had to restrict her intake while others didn't.

She had been to a dinner with her husband and two other couples. While she had been very sensible in what she ate, she felt a little aggrieved to see the other two couples "stuffing themselves" with food during the meal.

This kind of unfairness feeling can be very sabotaging for a weight loss programme. If you feel that you're suffering while everyone else is enjoying themselves, this can put off even the most committed person.

Luckily, in most cases, all you need to do is scratch the surface of these stories to see the reality.

In this case, of the four other people at dinner, three of them were overweight. Of course, if you're willing to be overweight then you can stuff yourself as much as you like.

I pointed out to my client that she could also eat like those people but she would have to put up with being overweight.

The remaining person, a woman in her 40s, was the client's very good friend. As it turns out, this woman ate much less during the week and was very active. In other words, this woman was practising balanced indulgence.

Either way, everyone must pay the piper. No one on this planet can continually eat heavy meals every day and not gain weight.

A caveat
Balanced indulgence does not mean skipping meals.

I have seen a few women who skipped meals as part of their attempt to lose weight.

This doesn't work, because as soon as you start skipping meals, you send panic signals to the body. Your body reacts by slowing your metabolism and holding on to fat stores. This is obviously counter-productive.

Continue to eat normally timed meals, but just reduce the amount you eat.

Eat what you want
It's therefore easy to eat what you want and enjoy life if you use balanced indulgence. As long as you compensate either before or after, you can enjoy more indulgent meals and still maintain a healthy weight.

Chapter 7 Summary

1. You can enjoy indulgent meals every now and then and not gain weight, if you balance your indulgence by cutting back either before or after the meal.
2. A normal eating pattern includes days when you eat more and days when you eat less. This means

you can have a "bad" day or even week and it shouldn't make much of a difference as long as you compensate for it.

3. Everyone must pay the piper. Anyone who eats too much will gain weight. The only way to dine out, eat a lot and not gain weight is through balanced indulgence.

8

EATING SLOWLY TO LOSE WEIGHT: TWENTY IDEAS TO SLOW DOWN EATING THAT DON'T INCLUDE "CHEW YOUR FOOD MORE"

W hat if I told you that there was a way to lose weight that required no expensive exercise equipment, complicated diet plans or calorie counting? And what if all it took was a few minutes extra at each meal?

In fact, research shows that if you slow down your speed of eating for three meals a day, you could end up eating two hundred fewer calories per day.[1] That adds up to 20 pounds over a year!

Next time you're at dinner with a few people (ideally around the same age as you), notice the speed at which different people at the table eat. You'll probably notice that the slimmest people at the table eat the slowest while the largest people eat the fastest.

Numerous research studies back this up: slim people eat slower than overweight people.[2,3,4] Eating faster means you eat more.[5] But not only does eating slowly mean that you eat less, it also means that you feel more satisfied after a meal.[6] And eating more slowly has been shown to lead to weight loss.[7]

This is why I tell my clients that when it comes to eating speed:

Slow = Slim

How does it work?
Why does slow eating of food correspond to being slimmer? The reason relates to how our bodies recognise that we are full. When our stomach starts to fill up with food or fluid, a signal is sent to the satiety (fullness) centre in our brain.[8]

Because it is quite a complicated system involving signals sent from your fat stores, intestine and stomach[9], it takes time for the signal to get through.

It is thought that people who eat slower allow enough time for the signal to reach their brain, and so they are able to feel full and therefore adjust their intake accordingly.[10]

How do you do it?
If you want the benefits of losing weight (feeling better, being healthier, having more energy) then eating slowly can be a valuable part of your approach. So the obvious advice people get given is to "just eat slower". Many people know this advice, but find it hard to implement. Why? Two reasons:

Firstly, it's hard to remember it. Most of my weight loss clients who try to eat more slowly find that despite their best intentions it's very easy to simply forget to do it. They'll get halfway through the meal and only then remember that they were meant to be eating slowly.

Secondly, the standard advice to slow down involves "chewing your food more". This is the ideal solution because it not only slows down eating but also aids in digestion.

But in my experience, most people struggle to do this. Some find chewing their food to a pulp to be quite unpleasant. Others find it boring. And it becomes less practical at functions or social occasions.

So eating slowly is good for you, but we need a more practical, sustainable solution than chewing more and we also need better ways to remember to do it.

Here are 20 ways to eat slower (that don't include chewing your food more):

1. At the beginning of starting any new behaviour, you need to clarify your motivation. In the case of eating slowly, you need to be convinced that it's worthwhile. If you're even half doubtful, it's unlikely that you'll follow through on your good intentions.

    This conviction that eating slowly is worthwhile must be tied in with your desire to lose weight. Make sure that you're absolutely convinced that adding a few minutes to your meal times will make you eat less.

    Look at the research yourself if it helps to convince you (in the notes section at the end of this book). Then try it out to see whether eating slowly makes a difference.

2. An important part of any behavioural programme is self-monitoring: keeping track of the behaviour. This way you can assess your current eating speed

and see your progress as you start eating more slowly. I get my clients to time their meals.

This alone can be very illuminating. When you time your meals, time only the main course, since meal times will vary depending on how many courses in your meal.

Another technique for assessing your eating speed is to compare yourself to others at the table.

3. You need to set aside the time to eat. Don't treat meal times as something that happens on the run, or something that you fit in between everything else in your life. Consciously try to make time for eating.

4. Drink water between bites. Having a sip of still or sparkling water between bites can slow down your eating. It also makes you feel full.

5. Talk a lot. You may not become that popular at dinner parties (depending on the quality of your dinner conversation) but talking a lot during a meal can really slow you down.

    We've probably all had experiences where we spoke a lot during a meal and then noticed that we'd hardly touched our food.

6. Use smaller utensils. You fit less food on smaller forks and knives each time you take a bite. This is an ingenious way of slowing down your eating.

7. Chopsticks works in the same way as using smaller utensils. The worse you are at using chopsticks, the slower your eating will be. I'm not sure how chopsticks work with eating steak, though.

8. Put your cutlery down between bites. This is a habit that is relatively easy to adopt.

9. Don't eat lunch in front of the computer. People who eat while multi-tasking slip into automatic or unconscious eating styles. While on your computer, it's easy to wolf down your food, and not even remember any of the individual bites.

10. Savour your food. This tip transcends slow eating. It's just a good tip full stop. Many of my clients talk about how when they're eating "bad" foods like ice cream, chocolates and sweets, they often eat them very quickly out of guilt.

    Instead, you should relish the taste of chocolate or ice cream when you do have it. Even with regular meals, if you're having something you enjoy then eat it slowly, taking time to revel in each bite.

    The more time food spends in the mouth means, the more exposure to the taste and enjoyment of the food, which helps you feel more satisfied and so you eat less.[11]

11. Don't eat while you walk. It's natural that when you're walking and eating you eat things faster. Don't do it.

12. Similar to eating in front of the computer, eating in front of the TV can make people eat faster and also do so on complete automatic pilot.

13. If you don't like food going cold partway through the meal (I don't) and that's why you eat fast, then why not serve less and take it straight from the original pot from where it will be warmer.

14. Or you can re-heat the meal partway through.

15. Or you can buy heat-retentive plates that keep your meal warm so that you can slow down.

16. If you struggle to slow down eating, then another alternative is to take a short pause before the end of the meal.

    Most people find that even a ten-minute break means that when they return to the rest of the meal they don't feel anywhere near as hungry as they would have if they'd kept ploughing through their food without a break.

17. Starting with something hot, like soup, forces you to slow down your eating.

18. Leave a reminder somewhere on the table, or wherever you eat your meals. This can be in the form of a brightly coloured piece of paper, or something else that's not usually placed there.

    One of my clients used to place a vase with flowers on it where she would usually put her plate. She would have to move the vase to put her plate down and that reminded her to slow down eating.

As with all reminders, you stop noticing them after two to three days, so you need to move them around.

19. Set an alarm to sound every few minutes during your meal to remind you to keep slowing down. Don't worry, you won't need this for the rest of your life, just as long as it takes to make it a habit.
20. Get someone else you live with to remind you. Better yet, try to make everyone you live with eat slowly with you.

You don't need to do all of these for every bite or every meal. But a combination would certainly help you to eat more slowly.

I don't have time to eat slowly
Many of my clients, when they first come and see me, are fast eaters. When I suggest they should slow down their eating, many of them bristle at the thought. Their response is often: "I have too much to do to waste time eating slowly." To which I say:

"Either spend a few more minutes at each meal, or spend many weeks trying to lose weight later."

While there are many ways to reduce your calorie intake, eating slowly is one that is both safe and healthy, and it can be very effective.

Chapter 8 Summary

1. Eating slowly means that you eat less and feel more satisfied.
2. For an investment of a few minutes extra per meal the payoff is huge. It's worth it.
3. The biggest obstacles are forgetting and thinking that chewing your food is the only way to do it.
4. Pick two to three of the twenty strategies and apply them to your life.

9

ENOUGH'S ENOUGH: FIGHTING YOUR BRAIN'S BAD DECISIONS ABOUT FOOD PORTIONS

What determines how much we eat? When you order food at a restaurant, prepare a meal at home or serve yourself food at a party, are you really able to make decisions that truly reflect your body's needs?

Although it would seem that a lifetime of eating should mean that we're able to see food and make accurate estimates of how much we need in order to feel satisfied and to cover our nutritional needs, the reality is that we're easily influenced and put off by the simplest of factors.

One of these factors is portion size.

Portion size tends to have a disproportionate effect on the amount we eat. Studies have shown that people who are given large portions of food tend to eat more than people who are given smaller portions.

In one study, where groups of men and women were given packets of crisps (potato chips) of different sizes, women ate 18 per cent more when portion size was doubled.[1]

In another study based on portions of macaroni cheese, when portion size doubled, people ate 30 per cent more.[2]

Why does portion size affect us so much?

Unit Bias
Part of it has to do with something called *unit bias*.[3] Unit bias means that people tend to unconsciously assume that whatever serving a food comes in is the optimal serving size for that food.

What this means is that if a chocolate bar comes in a particular size, we think that's probably a good serving. Never mind that the chocolate company came up with the size and it has nothing to do with our own needs.

What this also means is that if the chocolate bar was half the size, we'd still assume it represented a serving size, and similarly if it was double the size.

Of course, this doesn't apply at the extremes. If the chocolate bar was 50 times bigger, you wouldn't eat the whole thing and assume it was a serving size but...you would eat more than if you'd been given the usual size.

Furthermore, if we look at average serving size over the last few decades, especially in the United States, we can see that what people consider to be an average serving has increased a lot, showing that there's no such thing as a standard serving size.

We seem to believe that no matter what the size of the portion is, it's the appropriate one. We don't give any thought as to whether the portion size truly represents our needs.

You can see this at work when you go to a restaurant. The chef or restaurant owner decides what the serving size is and gives it to you. And you eat it, regardless of how much is there.

How did the chef know how much you needed to feel satisfied? Of course the chef didn't. Let's face it, sometimes even when we serve ourselves we get it wrong. And yet we obediently finish whatever is given to us by others.

The Completion Compulsion
As well as *unit bias*, the other part of the equation is the *completion compulsion*. The completion compulsion[4]

describes how we feel the need to complete a meal, regardless. We treat meals and other foods as units and we feel compelled to complete the unit of food. This is due to a number of different reasons.

The most obvious one is childhood conditioning. Almost all children are told to finish everything on their plates. It becomes ingrained in our minds that we must finish everything regardless of how much is there.

Part of this is the guilt induction that it's bad to waste food, hence we should finish everything (more about this later).

We may also finish everything on our plate because we find the food tempting, even if it's more than we need. We like the taste and because it's sitting in front of us we can't help but finish it.

The brain's food blind spot

If only the brain was able to look at food, see how many calories it contained and make a decision about how much to eat based on that calculation. Sadly, the amount we eat has almost nothing to do with calories.

For instance, if you were to go for a dinner where you had a choice between eating two massive plates of lettuce or a quarter of a plate of fries, which one would leave you feeling more full?

Most people would feel quite full after eating two massive plates of lettuce. Almost certainly the quarter plate of fries wouldn't fill them up either.

But the fact is, there are many more calories in the quarter plate of fries than in the two full plates of lettuce.

The brain and your fullness signals don't work on calories. They rely on volume (and the unit bias I mentioned earlier) to figure out how much to eat.

Experiments done by Dr. Brian Wansink at Cornell University's Food and Brand Laboratory have confirmed that much of our estimate of how much fulfils us comes from visual estimates of volume.

Also, because of unit bias, we estimate what a portion size is, and then feel satisfied from it.

A classic experiment in which he hooked up tubes pumping soup into bowls showed that most people kept drinking as long as the bowl was still full.

One participant even commented on how filling the soup was, because he had drunk two pints of it.

In this case, the participant was being compelled by the completion compulsion to keep going, hence overriding his natural feelings of fullness.[5]

Dr. Wansink also showed that increasing plate size can make people serve themselves more food.

In a study he ran, people who were given larger bowls dished out 31 per cent more ice cream than people who were given smaller bowls.

In addition, people who were given larger bowls and larger spoons with which to serve the ice cream ate 57 per cent more.[6]

The upshot of this? Buy smaller plates and smaller serving spoons.

As I tell my clients:

"A small plate = a small waist."

So there isn't a specific amount that we need to eat to feel full. We use volume and unit bias and we eat (complete) whatever we're given.

We're also creatures of habit. We may have a usual amount that we serve ourselves. Sometimes, without thinking about it, our portion size gets larger and larger. This will often mirror a rise in weight.

Other times we maintain our portion sizes from younger days, even though our body requirements aren't as much any more.

So what do we do about this?

Overcoming your brain biases and reducing portion size
Here are nine tips to help you overcome your brain biases and reduce portion size:

1. The first thing you need to do is to take control of your portion sizes.

    Instead of becoming a victim of the food company or the chef at the restaurant, take ownership of how much you eat. Don't just go for the default.

2. Aim to eat 5 - 10 per cent less. Serve yourself less. Experiment with this. See how much you can reduce without noticing a difference.

3. Try to overcome completion compulsion. If you're full partway through a meal, then stop.

    Get away from the habit of finishing food regardless of fullness. Some people find this relatively easy to do. Others struggle, because they feel like they're defying those wise words from their mother to finish everything on their plate.

I had a client who'd grown up in the post-war years in England where there was food rationing. She'd had it ingrained in her mind that to "waste" food by not eating what was on her plate was inexcusable. Interestingly enough, it only took her a few weeks to change this.

4. If you really feel you can't leave food on your plate, then just serve yourself less.

5. If you can, try to share food with someone else; for example, instead of ordering a full dessert, just split it with a friend.

6. At home, serve yourself food on smaller plates and drinks in long, thin glasses.

7. Break foods down to the smallest serving possible.

When eating pre-packaged foods like chocolate bars, pick the smallest size you can (ideal) or snap the bar in half and either give that portion away to someone else (also ideal), throw it away (less ideal), or keep it for another day (less ideal also).

8. If you want to portion off food, do it early.

Rather than eat 80 per cent of the chips and then sit there trying to resist the remaining 20 per cent at the end of the meal, portion off the 20 per cent early. Either give it to someone else or throw it away. Do this with food served on your plate too.

9. Don't eat from the bag. Eating crisps (chips) from the bag is a recipe for disaster. The larger the bag, the more unit bias and completion compulsion kick in, and next thing you know, the bag has been finished.

Food wastage

A few people might find it offensive to think that I'm advising people to leave food on their plate. Of course, if you can avoid it, you should always aim to have only what you need on the plate to begin with.

But in situations where you have no control over how much is served to you (for example, in a restaurant), then I don't see how you're helping anyone by continuing to eat something even after you're full.

If we consider the restaurant example in more detail, we can see that once food is put on your plate at a restaurant it's never going to be eaten by someone else (you hope!).

In other words, once the food was put on your plate, it was used up. Whether you put it in your mouth or it ends up in the waste doesn't change that fact.

As I tell my clients:

"It's either in the waste or on your waist."

Your purpose isn't to clean up leftover food. You're not a better person simply because you finished everything on your plate.

If you really feel strongly about not wasting food, go into the kitchen and advise the chef exactly how much you need. (Advisory note: this won't go down too well with most chefs.)

This also applies to packaged food. If you buy a chocolate bar and you feel full halfway through, you're not doing the world any favours by finishing it off to avoid wasting it. Sharing it with someone else is always an option. So is keeping it for later.

But don't kid yourself that eating something is a way of not wasting food.

The food was "wasted" the moment it was prepared. If you don't eat it or you do eat it, if it was surplus to requirements, it was a waste.

And why is putting it in your mouth after the point at which you felt full NOT wasting it? Don't kid yourself that forcing extra food into your body isn't just another form of wastage.

Take Control

Portion size represents one of those areas of your diet where you could potentially be giving up control of your health to other people. You become a victim of the environment.

The chef at the restaurant becomes the person that decides how much you need to satisfy your appetite. The people at the chocolate company decide how much chocolate you should have as a snack.

It is also one of those areas where you can cut down the amount you eat without jeopardising any enjoyment. If you stop eating the moment it stops being enjoyable, you are, by definition, maximising your enjoyment and minimising the calories.

Don't underestimate the difference that leaving a few extra (unsatisfying) bites can have over a year. And it's a prime opportunity to live well without the nasty consequences of being overweight.

Chapter 9 Summary

1. Portion size exerts a huge influence over how much you eat (even though you'd think that it logically shouldn't).

2. We have a tendency to assume that whatever serving size we're given is the appropriate one, and finish it.
3. Don't let arbitrary serving sizes control you.
4. Experiment with portion sizes. Use the different strategies provided to reduce your portion sizes to the amount you actually need, not the "usual", habitual amount you eat or an amount decided by someone else.

10

EXERCISE: IS IT AS IMPORTANT AS YOU THINK?

Most of us know that exercise is a vital part of a healthy lifestyle. There are so many positives related to being active every day. But for many people, especially as they get older, their main motivation for exercise is to lose weight.

Many women feel that the one thing preventing them from losing weight is that they're not doing enough exercise.

Even women who are quite physically active berate themselves, thinking that the key to losing weight for them would be to push themselves even harder at the gym.

But the fact is, it's very difficult for women to lose weight with exercise alone. Let me repeat this, because it's very important and most women don't hear it the first time. For a woman to lose weight, sweating it out at the gym *without* changing what she eats is a recipe for failure.

> For women, exercise alone is NOT enough to lose weight.

Men can often just focus on exercise to lose weight (although this is a risky strategy, as I'll explain later), but for women (especially as they get older) this isn't the case.

This explains why many women tell me that they went to the gym five times a week for a month and didn't lose a pound of weight. (Let's set aside the fact that weight alone is a poor indicator of health.)

When I tell women that exercise alone isn't enough to lose weight, they don't believe me, even if their own personal experience seems to confirm it. After all, it's drummed into us how important exercise is for losing weight. Many GPs (family doctors), when faced with an overweight patient and limited options for what to do, will tell them to join a gym.

Given all this, it seems crazy, even improper to suggest that exercise doesn't make a difference for weight loss. But that's not what I'm saying. I'm saying exercise *alone* isn't effective for weight loss.

If you're a woman who's exercising regularly but still eating the same amount, you'll struggle to lose weight. You need to also change how much you're eating.

Let me give you a scenario; see whether you can guess the outcome:

Let's say we took 131 women (this scenario is based on an actual research study[1]) and made 87 of them exercise regularly and the remainder (44) do no exercise at all.

And let's say for the first group that was exercising, we made them exercise for forty-five minutes a day, five days a week for sixteen months.

I don't need to tell you, that's an impressive amount of exercise. It's important to note that both groups ate their usual diet throughout the time.

So what do you think would happen? Which group would lose the most weight? How much weight do you think they would have lost?

Well, for a start, more than half of the exercisers (46 of the 87) dropped out of the study.

When you consider the commitment of exercising five days a week for sixteen months, that's not so surprising.

Only 11 of the 44 non-exercisers dropped out. Again, not surprising that fewer people dropped out of the non-exercise group.

So how much weight did the exercise group lose? Well, actually they didn't lose any weight at all. In fact they gained about 0.6 kilograms (one pound).

Let me just repeat that: women who exercised for forty-five minutes a day, five days a week for sixteen months gained one pound. Other studies have shown similar results to these.[2,3]

Now, you might think that one explanation for this was that while their weight was the same, their physique may have changed. They may have been more muscular and toned.

But measurements of fat-free mass, showed that there was no significant change in the physical make-up of the participants.

So if women exercising five days a week for sixteen months can't lose weight, then it seems clear that pushing yourself to exercise more isn't the solution.

So what's the solution? The solution is that if you're a woman serious about losing weight:

1. You need to combine exercise with dietary adjustments. **You must change how much you eat** in order to achieve weight loss. There are no two ways about this.
2. If you're doing a lot of exercise, don't beat yourself up that it still isn't enough.

Some people have misinterpreted this message as being "Don't bother exercising". But this is the wrong conclusion to make.

Let's not forget that exercise is of course about more than just weight loss. Exercise has a vast number of other benefits.[4]

Whenever I read a list of benefits of exercise I'm always reminded of those "health tonics" they used to sell in the 19th century that promised to help almost any bodily ailment.

In that case, it was more of a case of creative marketing, but with exercise, the benefits are genuine. Exercise can:

1. Help your heart function better and reduce the risks of you having a heart attack.

2. Reduce the chance of you having a stroke. A stroke occurs when the blood supply to a part of your brain is stopped. It can result in paralysis of a side of your body or an inability to speak, amongst other effects.

3. Reduce your blood pressure. High blood pressure makes you more likely to have a heart attack or a stroke.

4. Lower cholesterol. There are two types of cholesterol that will often be reported in the blood tests that you get. One is LDL, which is characterised as "bad" cholesterol, and the other, HDL, is characterised as "good" cholesterol. Exercise helps increase the levels of good cholesterol, HDL.

5. Reduce your chance of developing type 2 diabetes. Exercise can also help with blood sugar levels if you're diabetic. Poorly controlled blood sugar levels can eventually cause damage to kidneys, arteries, nerves and eyes.

6. Prevent lower back and joint pain, or make it better if you already have it.

7. Reduce the chance of developing low bone density (osteoporosis). People with osteoporosis are more likely to suffer bone fractures.

8. Reduce the chance of developing colon cancer and breast cancer (especially after a woman's periods stop).

9. Reduce your chance of developing depression.

In addition, people who are active:

1. Feel better about themselves.
2. Feel less anxious.
3. Sleep better.
4. Have better concentration.
5. Feel more satisfied with life.

Just reading this list of benefits makes me want to go out and exercise.

But getting back to weight loss, exercise has also been shown to be effective for *maintaining* weight loss.

In that scenario I described above, the group of women who did no exercise did worse than those who did exercise. While the exercising group gained 0.6 kilograms, the non-exercising group gained three kilograms. That's almost half a stone.

In other words, if you want to remain at a particular weight then exercise is helpful. This may not seem like a priority when you're overweight, but **it should be** a priority because:

1. Once you lose weight, you want to be able to maintain it. If not, you'll be locked into a cycle of weight loss and gain: so-called yo-yo dieting.

2. If you don't lose weight but you also can't maintain
    your weight as it is, you'll continue to gain weight,
    like the non-exercising group in the above study.

So, exercise may not be useful in the initial stages
of weight loss for women, but it becomes much more
important in maintaining the gains you've made.

Why is exercise not effective in women compared
to men? It's probably related to muscle mass. Men have
more muscle mass so when they're active they burn
more calories.

So men might be thinking that they're on easy street
here. They *can* lose weight through exercise.[1]

Men often say that they'll eat whatever they want
(more than they need) because they can rely on heavy
exercise to keep them on track. But relying on exercise
alone is a dangerous idea.

What happens if you get injured? What happens if
you're unwell? What happens if you can't make it to the
gym for a few weeks?

These things happen, and men who rely purely on
extreme exercise to keep them in shape soon start gaining weight after they stop exercising.

Diet is better than exercise for losing weight, but the ideal combination for weight loss is a combination of the two.[5]

In the National Weight Loss Registry (of people who have achieved and maintained weight loss) which was mentioned in Chapter 3, 90 per cent of people who had lost and maintained weight loss had combined intake reduction (eating less) with exercise to lose weight. Nine per cent had used intake reduction alone and only 1 per cent used exercise alone.[6]

The problem for many clients I see is that they're not particularly keen on exercise.

In fact, it's estimated that only 29 per cent of women (and 39 per cent of men) in the UK get their recommended amount of exercise in a week[7] (the recommended amount of physical activity per week is 30 minutes of moderate activity, five times per week[7]).

Part of the problem is that people go about starting an exercise habit in the wrong way.

Let me give you an example. One of my clients (before I'd met her) had tried to improve her physical fitness by waking at 5.30 each morning and running two miles. She managed it for two days in a row before the weather turned bad and her snooze button trumped her morning exercise routine.

This story is very common, but why does it happen? Because the behaviour was too much, too soon. It wasn't part of my client's routine, and need I mention, she didn't really enjoy it.

Instead of the "shock and awe" approach, the solution is to go for a "think big but start small" approach. Instead of aiming for two miles a day in the early morning, my client could have aimed for a five-minute walk at lunchtime.

Now you might think that's ridiculous. No one is going to get fit from five minutes a day. But that would be missing the point.

In the beginning, it's not about how far you walk or run, it's about developing the habit of doing exercise.

By settling for a small amount to begin with, you're getting success under your belt. Because it's not unpleasant, you'll feel less resistance to going again the next day.

Because it's only five minutes, you can't use the "I've got no time" excuse. The exercise is much less likely to interfere with your schedule.

This five minutes repeated over a longer period of time will turn into a habit. As it becomes more ingrained, you can increase the amount of time you exercise. *Et voilà*, you're now exercising consistently.

Instead of small two-day bursts of iron-man/-woman type activity that never get you anywhere, you're now a once-a-day exerciser.

What about people who have such an ingrained habit that they never miss a day of exercise? How do they develop that?

Well, let me ask you a question. Do you think that these people are motivated to exercise by all the amazing benefits of physical activity? Do they wake up and think how good doing exercise is going to make them feel? Is that what keeps them going day to day?

No. Surprisingly, for people who can't miss going to the gym, this isn't their primary motivator.

Of course, overall they love the positive benefits, but when it's 6.30 in the morning and it's cold outside, the thing that gets them out of bed is thinking about how they'll feel if they *don't* go.

It's called anticipated regret.[8] They think about how bad they'll feel if they don't manage to exercise that day.

And so if you aren't active enough, you need to replicate their motivation. You need to emphasise and notice the difference between when you do go and when you don't go.

The other mistake I see many people making is that they choose the wrong type of exercise. Whatever activity you choose, don't take a short-term approach.

The bike you love to hate

Let me give you an example with a client called Sandra. Sandra had been my client for a few weeks and was starting to lose weight. She was walking to and from work every day, which I thought was excellent.

But during our weekly consultation, she suddenly said at one of the sessions that she needed to do more. So she was going to buy a stationary bike and cycle on that for half an hour a day.

And so I asked her, "Is this something you think you'll be doing in six years' time?"

She said, "Probably not."

"Do you think you'll still be doing it in six months?"

"Maybe not."

"In six weeks?"

"No."

"Why not?"

"Because I hate cycling."

This sounds ridiculous, but so many people will start exercise routines doing things that they can barely tolerate, and then wonder why exercise goes out the window at the first sign of an excuse.

If you're going to do anything to manage your weight, do things that you know you can do forever, for the rest of your life. That applies equally to exercise as to eating behaviours.

What if you don't like exercise?
So what happens if you're one of those people who just doesn't like exercise? For many of my clients the word exercise conjures up images of scary gyms, exercise equipment, sweatiness and discomfort. If you're one of these people, no problem.

The research evidence shows that when it comes to managing your weight, incorporating more activity into your daily life can be just as effective as formal exercise.[9,10]

Incorporating more exertion into your life is called lifestyle activity. It means doing what you normally do as part of your activities of daily living, but trying to make yourself more active at the same time.

Here are some examples of ways to increase lifestyle activity:

- Housework, including hanging laundry, sweeping, vacuuming, scrubbing floors
- Gardening, including mowing lawns, pruning, weeding, planting trees
- Five-minute walks
- Playing with your children or grandchildren
- Parking the car a bit further away from where you want to go
- Making a rule that for any stairs under five floors, you take the stairs
- Walking around while talking on the phone
- Walking the dog
- Getting off the bus one stop early and walking
- Walking instead of taking the tube one stop to transfer

- Walking up and down the platform while waiting for the train or tube
- Arranging to meet friends and go walking
- Having meetings while walking
- Walking down the hall to speak to someone at work instead of emailing or calling them
- Dancing to music at home
- Pacing and stretching while watching TV

A good way to start applying lifestyle changes to your daily activities is to keep a log. Break up bursts of activity into small segments. Ten-minute bursts are enough.[11,12,13] Each time you do an activity, write it down. Aim for at least three ten-minute bursts per day.

Chapter 10 Summary

1. Don't rely on exercise alone to lose weight.
2. Stop blaming yourself if you're exercising every day and still not losing weight.
3. You need to combine increased activity with eating changes for maximum results.
4. Instead of overwhelming yourself, start small and build up the habit.
5. Use the power of anticipated regret to get motivated. Notice how bad you feel when you don't exercise compared to when you do.

6. Whatever you decide to do, make sure it's something you would do for the long term.
7. Incorporate activity into your daily life.

11

"BECAUSE IT WAS THERE": HOW YOUR ENVIRONMENT AFFECTS WHAT YOU EAT AND WHAT TO DO ABOUT IT

Why is the number of overweight and obese people in our society so high? Why is the number increasing every year?

The number one culprit has to be our environment. Not only does our environment promote sedentary behaviour, but everywhere we go we're surrounded by temptation to eat things that we shouldn't and to eat more than we know we need.

When you go out of the house, you're surrounded by shops that serve high-calorie, energy-dense foods. Advertisements at home and outside make eating those foods feel like a matter of necessity. Our friends all go out and eat a lot. Our lifestyle is built around convenience and eating high-calorie foods.

This isn't a rally against modernity or our current lifestyles. This is just to say that this is the environment that we live in. Plenty of remarkable people are trying to make changes on a community and global level, but on a more immediate level, if you're waiting for the world to change and prevent you from gaining weight, you're going to be sorely disappointed.

You need to take responsibility for your environment.

The Mount Everest strategy

We make decisions based on what we see in our environment. And these decisions are largely a result of how we structure our lives and how we enable our environment to have an effect on our lives.

The English mountaineer George Mallory was once asked why he wanted to climb Mount Everest and he famously replied: "Because it's there."

There are some people who use the Mount Everest strategy with food: "Why did you eat that piece of cake?" "Because it was there."

One of my clients once told me that offering her food was like "pushing against an open door". The point is, we're hardwired to be like this. When food is presented to us, we're naturally inclined to want it. And the more fat and sugar in the food, the more we desire it.

Our ancestors couldn't afford to be so picky with food. If they didn't eat when they had the opportunity, they didn't know when the next meal would be available.

If food is in front of you, you have to make a decision as to whether to eat it or not. And if you like the food, your mind will always tend towards thinking yes.

I teach my clients to get around this in a number of ways, but the most obvious is to avoid the decision in the first place. If the food isn't in front of you, you don't have to make this decision.

In behavioural psychology this is called stimulus control. The environment acts as a stimulus to perform a certain behaviour. If you modify or remove the stimulus you can change or stop the behaviour.

If we make some small changes to our environment, we can reduce our exposure to the food to begin with. This means the "should I eat this?" question never comes up.

An example from Dr. Brian Wansink at Cornell University's Food and Brand Laboratory illustrates how destructive the ready availability of food can be.

In an experiment made famous in his excellent book *Mindless Eating*[1], secretaries in a workplace were given a bowl full of chocolates but there were four different placement conditions.

- On their desk with a clear lid on the bowl so the chocolates were close-by and visible.
- On their desk with an opaque lid on the bowl so the chocolates were close-by and not visible.
- On a filing cabinet six feet away with a clear lid (far away and visible).
- On a filing cabinet six feet away with an opaque lid (far away and not visible).

The researchers monitored how many chocolates the secretaries ate in a day and rotated the placement at the end of each week (for a total of four weeks).

The results showed that when the bowl was on their desk and visible, the secretaries had on average eight chocolates a day.

When the bowl was on the desk but had an opaque lid (out of sight) they ate five a day.

When the bowl was on the filing cabinet six feet away (further away) and the chocolate visible they took six chocolates a day.

And when the bowl was both further away and the contents not visible they only ate three a day[2]

This showed that when the chocolates were in sight, the secretaries ate more. And when the chocolates were placed further away, they ate less.

In other words, when the food is in front of us, we must continually ask the question, "Should I have this?" And even if we give in once every ten times that we ask the question, that's enough to cause a significant increase in intake over a long period of time.

If we take the example of the secretaries, eating eight chocolates a day contributes two hundred extra calories per day. If all else remained the same, it could mean up to ten to fourteen pounds weight gained in a year. It is truly amazing how such small changes can have such a large effect.

The desk smorgasbord
If you want to manage your weight successfully, you must learn to control your environment.

Let me give you an example of one of my clients. Let's call her Carol.

Carol worked in an office and she mentioned that she often snacked at her desk. That's not unusual. But on further questioning, it sounded like she had set up her workspace like a corporate buffet table.

She had crackers, dips, chocolates, donuts and biscuits. It was all on her table and, like the secretaries in the research study I mentioned earlier, she was a victim to their availability. She was snacking throughout the day.

When we spoke about this, Carol felt that it would be too difficult to stop snacking altogether. Instead, we decided that she could have whatever she wanted, but she had to locate the food elsewhere.

At her workplace, the kitchen was downstairs. So I said to her that she could have all the food she wanted on the proviso that she had to go downstairs and eat in the kitchen. She couldn't bring food back up to her desk.

That one change made a world of difference to Carol's snacking. This lack of convenience or availability – the fact that she had to make the effort of going downstairs to snack – meant that she cut back considerably.

She ended up losing over 20 pounds of weight, and I'm sure the reduced snacking at work contributed a lot to that.

Looking at your environment
Let's work through all the areas in your life and see where there is scope for making changes. (Please note that while travel and eating out are part of your environment, I have covered these separately in Chapter 14: Having a Life.)

The obvious place to start is at home.

- How is your home set up for food?
- What foods do you keep at home?
- Are there lots of snacks?
- Are there lots of high-fat, high-sugar foods? The more snacks and foods there are in your house, the more likely you'll be tempted to eat them.
- Is there a shop nearby that you're able to access easily to buy snacks and high-fat, high-sugar foods? Do you need to make a rule that you no longer visit that shop?
- Do you buy in bulk? When people buy in bulk, they buy more than they need, and end up eating more just to get value out of the purchase. The amount of money you might save will be outweighed by the effects on your health.

- Do you eat in all rooms of the house? An effective strategy is to only eat in one room of the house. This eliminates snacking in the bedroom, or while watching TV.
- Do you snack in front of the TV? Automatic eating while watching TV is a prime cause of unnecessary eating. Most of the time you don't even taste what you're eating while engrossed in your favourite programme.

  As we've discussed, if you get neither health benefits nor enjoyment (taste) from something (the magic margin – see Chapter 4) then it's time to stop it.

  Eliminate eating in front of the TV from your life and you'll notice a big change in the amount you eat.
- What is your home roadmap like? Do you often walk past the kitchen or the fridge?

  I've had clients who ate very little during meals, but because they were often walking past the fridge at home they grazed a lot. This was enough to account for significant weight gain over several years.

Travel

Do you often drive or walk past places where there is temptation?

Simply walking past a cake store or a chocolate shop or even a fast food restaurant can be tempting. If you do this twice a day, for every five times you walk past you might make the decision to eat there once, and that's enough to add a significant amount of calories to your life over a year or so.

The irony is that if you hadn't walked past there, you wouldn't have noticed anything or missed not having it. This is classic unnecessary eating.

Change your travel route to avoid unnecessary temptation.

Work

- Do you keep a lot of food on your desk?
  Like Carol, keeping food there might seem like a guilty pleasure that brightens up the work day. That's fine; you can still have those rewards if you must, but keep them away from your desk so you're not continually tempted.
- Do you have access to lots of food at work, such as in vending machines? This may require that you make a rule for yourself that you don't use it, or you only use it once a day or once a week.

- Is there generally unhealthy food at work? Many workplaces only have unhealthy food there. This can be difficult, but you need to come up with some way to avoid it.
- Bring your own snacks and lunch. Or make a rule to get food from elsewhere in your lunch break.
- Do you have workmates who often eat tempting, unhealthy foods? See Chapter 13 on obligation eating.

If your health truly is important to you and you want to get the benefits of losing weight, you need to make some changes. And one of these involves taking control of your environment.

The best part of taking control of your environment is that you're able to retain the same level of enjoyment of food, with just small changes. Controlling your environment is much more powerful and easier to do than relying on willpower.

Chapter 11 Summary

1. Your environment has a massive effect on your eating patterns.
2. If you control your environment, you'll make it much easier to lose weight.

3. Do an audit of your food environment. Are you simply eating things because they are there?
4. Make changes to ensure that your environment is clear and free from undue influences.

12

DANGER FOOD: DO YOU HAVE
TO CUT OUT ALL THE FOODS
YOU LOVE IN ORDER TO LOSE
WEIGHT? NO!

When you decide to lose weight, it can be tempting to think that the first step is to cut out those "bad" foods out of your diet. This appears to make sense, since it was the chocolate, the crisps (chips), the bread and the biscuits that got you to where you are today. It stands to reason that they all must go.

This is very closely related to the all-or-nothing approach perpetuated by most diets. You either follow the diet perfectly (cutting out all the foods you crave) or you're not on the diet at all.

I frequently meet people who are trying to lose weight before getting married. Their usual habits involve eating large portions of high-calorie foods and doing no exercise, hence the reason they're overweight.

And in most cases their plan to lose weight involves eating nothing but "healthy" foods and exercising every day. An honourable plan, but one with a very low likelihood of success.

As I've discussed earlier, drastic changes are a sure way to failure.

The more difficult it is to stick to a diet, the less likely it is that you will. If you want to move from what you eat now to a healthier version that helps you lose weight, I recommend going about it in a way that maximises your chances of success.

The more difficult it is to stick to a diet, the less likely it is that you will.

You maximise your chances by making things easy. The easier your plan is to follow, the more likely it is that you'll persist.

And if you deny yourself all the foods you like, that deprivation alone will drive your cravings and make success ever more elusive.

Because of this, I generally don't tell my clients what they should and shouldn't eat. I nudge them towards healthier choices, but no food is ever forbidden.

But there is one food that is an exception. Is it chocolate? Is it pizza? Is it crisps (potato chips)? Well, actually it depends. The food I recommend cutting out is called a *danger food* and it varies from person to person. What is a danger food for you may not be a danger food for me.

What makes something a danger food is that it accounts for disproportionately more calories in your diet than other foods. This is because it's both a high-calorie food and because you eat more of it than other foods.

Another characteristic of danger foods is that if you start eating them you can't stop. For example, you say you're only going to have a scoop of ice cream and end up polishing off the entire tub.

Danger foods also create a pattern of desiring that food every day. For example, when you have a piece of chocolate after dinner one day then you have the craving for it the next day too.

I know about danger foods first hand, because for a couple of years my danger food was crisps (chips). The more I ate them, the more I wanted to eat them. They started creeping in from a few with lunch to a between-meals snack to an after-dinner snack too.

With most foods, you can be moderate. By practising moderation, you can have whatever you want, as long as you watch the amounts. With danger foods, this isn't possible. You can't eat the danger food in moderation because one leads to another and then another.

The beauty of the danger food approach is that instead of removing every single "bad" food from your life, you can concentrate on only one type of food.

In other words, it maximises the benefit for minimum pain. When you focus on only one type of food that adds lots of calories to your diet, you'll see results relatively quickly. And research shows that people who see results sooner are more likely to stick with a programme of weight loss.[1]

Applying this to your life

On a practical level, what does this mean?

Let's look at an example.

Diane enjoys eating chocolates, crisps and biscuits. On a regular diet, Diane would be instructed to stop eating all of them. Poor Diane.

This kind of all-or-nothing approach makes Diane's weight loss efforts seem very harsh and she's unlikely to persist for very long.

Even if Diane is able to persist for the time it takes to lose weight, then what? Does she start eating all of her favourite foods again? Or does she never eat them again?

If she starts again, she'll likely begin to gain weight. If she doesn't eat them at all, she'll be miserable. And if she tries something in between, how does she know what the right amount is?

But taking a different approach, what if Diane identified chocolate as her danger food.

Chocolate is her danger food because not only does she eat more of it, but once she starts she finds it hard to stop. Therefore, instead of not eating crisps, biscuits and chocolate, the best idea for Diane would be to just focus on not eating chocolate.

One change is easier

Think about it. Which is easier? Cutting all "bad" foods out, or just one thing? Of course, cutting out one thing is easier. And what you find is that simply cutting out the chocolate might mean 300 calories less per day. This adds up to a lot of weight over a year (maybe up to 30 pounds).

The one change (as long as everything else stays the same) can sometimes be enough to kick-start a new weight loss effort. And it's so much easier than trying to do everything at once.

Know thy enemy

While reading this, you may have been able to identify your danger food immediately. For others it takes some thought.

If you aren't sure what your danger food is, then your food diary is your ally. Observe your food patterns.

Are there foods that make an appearance one day, and then continue appearing daily for several days afterwards? Or are there particular high-calorie foods that you always eat at the same time every day?

Are there foods you instinctively know that you can't resist? Sometimes your danger food can be replaced with an alternative that's not as moreish (makes you want to eat more).

For example, one of my clients replaced milk chocolate with dark chocolate because she found it harder to eat large amounts of dark chocolate compared to milk chocolate.

Sometimes you might feel that your danger food is alcohol. Certainly this is possible, but alcohol is different in that people can get physically dependent on alcohol.

Dependence means that you need increasing amounts to get the same effect, and when you try to cut back you start to get withdrawal symptoms. If you suspect that you're dependent on alcohol and want to do something about it, it's best to consult your GP / family doctor.

How to cut out your danger food
When you identify your danger food, don't try to cut it out immediately.

Make a schedule to slowly reduce the amount you eat over a few weeks (depending on how much you're eating now). And try to stick to the schedule.

Don't expect rapid progress straight away. These are ingrained habits, and it may take some time to adjust.

Pitfalls to avoid

- Don't try to cut two danger foods at the same time. This will feel too depriving and unpleasant and will therefore sabotage your efforts. Take things easy.
- Don't make the mistake of replacing your danger food with something even worse.

    One of my clients replaced a chocolate habit with granola bars. That was until she realised that she was eating three granola bars and that still didn't quite seem to scratch the itch of her craving. Three granola bars contain many more calories than a few squares of chocolate.
- Don't cut out your danger food and then let it creep back in. Some people will cut out a danger food and then start saying things like: "I'm allowed to have it once in a while."
- This once in a while soon turns into every day and then you're back with the same danger food problem again.
- Try to avoid keeping the danger food at home. It will act as a regular temptation. If you absolutely have to keep some at home (for example, for your children or grandchildren),

make sure it's out of sight and preferably in a separate cupboard to one that you routinely use.

— If the danger food creeps back in, don't feel bad. Just cut it back again. The fact that you did it once makes you more likely to succeed again.

Chapter 12 Summary

1. Your danger food is a food that contributes more calories than others and becomes something that you can't stop eating.
2. Instead of cutting out all bad foods, if you concentrate on your danger food, you can get maximum effect with minimum pain.
3. When you decide / find out what your danger food is, don't stop eating it immediately, but scale back gradually.
4. Another strategy is to replace the danger food with something similar that doesn't set up cravings and doesn't add as many calories.

13

"I DIDN'T WANT TO OFFEND THEM": HOW TO STOP EATING FOR OTHERS

"Whenever I go to my friend's house, she's always so insistent that I eat a lot. I feel it's so rude to refuse, but I end up eating much more than I wanted to."

Obligation eating, when you eat because you're scared of offending the person serving food, can have a big impact on your weight. For some of my clients it's one of the major contributors to their excess eating.

Given the negative impact that being overweight can have on your health, confidence, feelings of attractiveness and other areas it seems almost ridiculous that people would risk all of this just for the sake of not offending others.

But it's the natural instinct for humans to stick with the crowd and not offend.

When our ancestors lived in tribes, not going along with the crowd was a very bad move.

If you offended or went against the group, you ran the risk of being rejected by the tribe. Being out of the tribe meant that you were alone in the wilderness without the protection of others.

In other words, expulsion from the group was the equivalent of a death sentence.

This is why we hate to be rejected, stand out as being different or go against the crowd.

We care about what other people think. Of course, these days being socially embarrassed or making a scene doesn't have life and death implications, but these deeply imbedded patterns still hold sway.

For some people, obligation eating isn't such a big problem. They only rarely go out for dinner, host a party or dine at someone else's house.

Others, though, may regularly be in situations where people are serving them food with the expectation that they eat it.

My clients have described a wide variety of situations where this can occur. The most common is overbearing family or friends who feel that hospitality means forcing food on their guests.

But I've also had clients who frequently attend official functions where they're the guest of honour and they felt a weight of expectation to be the good guest and eat up.

What do we fear when we think of refusing food that someone offers us?

1. That they'll think we didn't like what they prepared.
2. That they'll think we're rude.

Sometimes you may not even get the choice of what you get served. Your plate will get loaded up with food and, not wanting to make a fuss or offend, you finish off the food, eating sometimes twice as much as you'd have normally eaten.

Although it's understandable that we're worried about what other people think, there can be a tendency to overestimate how much people care about us or what we're eating.

In some cases, even the host/hostess feels obliged to fuss and make sure you eat more, whether or not they care about it or not. Many cultures around the world feel this is a necessity.

Of course, the same people who force food down your throat are unlikely to be by your side when your excess weight leads to you having a heart bypass operation.

And this is the way you need to look at it. Is the risk of offending someone really worth endangering your health, as well as all the other negatives of being overweight or obese?

The cognitive therapist Judith Beck calls these people "food pushers".[1]

Food pushers also sometimes have nefarious aims. It's not unheard of for people to want to make others eat excessively because it makes them feel better about themselves.

Needless to say, this kind of behaviour shouldn't be tolerated. There are other ways of helping someone build their self-esteem that don't involve endangering your own health. And the sad thing is that often the food pushers are close family or friends, which is why you must be extra-vigilant.

Do They Really Care?
Often we mistakenly assume that people are truly pre-occupied with how much we eat.

One of my clients, let's call her Mary, had a group of friends with whom she would frequently go out for dinner. At these dinners, Mary felt the responsibility to be the life and soul of the party.

In her mind, part of this responsibility included eating and drinking a lot. Reading this now, it might seem quite apparent to you that being the life and soul of the party doesn't necessarily mean eating a lot, but this just serves to illustrate how much of our behaviour is driven by unconscious (and often wrong) assumptions.

Because being the life and soul of the party was part of her identity with that group, Mary felt that she would be letting the side down if she ate less. It would cause consternation and distress amongst her dining companions. It would almost be like she was betraying them.

After we had a lengthy discussion, Mary saw that the association between being the life and soul of the party and eating large amounts was illogical. But even then she struggled to make the change, because she didn't want to let down her friends. After all, their enjoyment of the evenings was very much dependent on her.

Despite these misgivings, I convinced Mary to try an experiment.

For the next dinner she had with these friends, she would only eat as much as she felt comfortable with. We prepared so that if her dining companions chided her or tried to force food on her, she had appropriate responses. And we agreed that if they became really distressed and pushy then she would give in and eat more.

She felt comfortable with the fact that not only could she give in to their pleas if it all became too intense, but also that this was a one-off experiment, so she could go back to being the life and soul at the next dinner.

Come the night of the big dinner, Mary had only one serving of the main course, no second servings and no dessert.

To her absolute shock, no one said a word. She wasn't even sure that anyone noticed.

While Mary was happy that she had managed to get through the meal without unnecessarily over-eating, she also felt quite upset. After all her internal conflict over the matter, as it turned out, *they didn't even care what she ate.*

She regretted all that extra food she had needlessly eaten over the years for the sake of her friends. But as I said to her, at least she had learnt this lesson now and not endured many more years of over-stuffed meals just for the sake of pleasing others.

I remember another client, Sarah, once refused a slice of someone's freshly baked cake. She felt so bad about it that when, a month later, she ran into the same person, she apologised. To Sarah's amazement, the woman didn't even remember that incident.

But don't take my word for it. Try it yourself. Refuse something that someone is pushing on you and then ask them about it in a week's time. They won't have a clue what you're talking about.

When I tell the story of Sarah, the occasional person says, "The woman was just being polite. She remembered and was probably deeply offended." Okay. So what if someone does take offence and remembers it forever more?

Although this scenario is highly unlikely, let's talk this through. Let's consider someone who really has so little going on in their life that they have to nurse a deep hatred of you for not stuffing yourself with as much food as they wanted you to have.

If you were allergic to peanuts, would it be reasonable for the host to force a peanut brownie down your throat? Should a person with peanut allergies endanger their life in order to avoid offending a sensitive host?

What about a vegetarian? Would anyone argue that a vegetarian should eat meat just to satisfy the host?

Some might say that peanut allergy is a matter of life and death and so transcends the petty needs of the host. But tell that to someone who's suffering life-threatening complications of obesity.

And not feeding meat to a vegetarian may be a matter of respecting people's values, but I think your health and the decisions you make to manage your weight are values too. They're crucial to your health, so you need to stand by them.

Fortunately, people are getting much more health conscious and acknowledge that being sensible about what you eat is good for your health.

So what should you say to people who try to push food on you?

Here are some suggestions for how to deal with people trying to push food on you:

- If it's a second serving of the main course or the dessert, say, "Thank you, but I'm full."
- If they push you further, you can say, "I'm at a really nice food level now, and if I eat more, I'll feel too full. As much as I'd love to."
- If they get a bit pushier you can say, "I don't mean to hurt your feelings, I'm just too full to enjoy anything more."

Obligation eating is a trap that you don't want to fall into. It's needless eating in the purest sense of the word. It's food that's neither necessary for sustenance nor, because you're eating it for someone else's sake, personally enjoyable.

Remember, every calorie you consume needlessly to avoid offence is a calorie that you have to work off later.

Chapter 13 Summary

1. Acknowledge the unconscious assumptions you have about doing what other people say.

2. Realise that most people who push food on you mostly don't really care whether you eat or not.

3. Know that even for the people who do care whether you eat or not, eating excessively and all the effects it may have on you and your health are really not worth it.

4. Be especially vigilant towards malicious food pushers.

5. Have some responses prepared earlier to politely but firmly deal with food pushers.

14

HAVING A LIFE: HOW TO EAT OUT, GO ON HOLIDAY AND STILL LOSE WEIGHT

"I can't go out for dinner tonight, darling, I'm trying to lose weight." Overheard words of a woman sitting in a cafe in Chelsea, London (sorry for eavesdropping).

As I've mentioned throughout this book, the easier you make things for yourself, the more likely it is that you'll stick to your weight loss plan.

By this reasoning, if you decide that part of your drive to lose weight includes suspending all the finer things in life, then you're making things much harder for yourself.

What is life without eating out, travelling and having fun?

Unfortunately, many diets ignore the fun side of life and simply give you a strict regime to follow. Some people can tolerate this for a short time, but then what? Will you never eat out again?

Your life will be much the poorer if you can't enjoy pleasures in life such as eating out or travelling. And for many people it's a fact of life that they eat out and travel a lot. For many of my clients, the reality is that most of their meals are eaten out of the home.

In other cases, I've had clients who've always managed to maintain their weight while in London, but as soon as they went on holiday they would gain around one to two pounds.

Multiply that over two to three holidays per year over five years and you see that holiday weight gain alone accounted for their excess weight.

If you want to maintain a lifestyle that includes socialising, eating out and travelling then you'll most likely struggle to lose weight on a standard diet.

Most of my clients who've successfully lost weight using my approach haven't fared so well with other approaches.

For instance, there are some weight loss programmes where they deliver set meals to your house. I don't know what they tell you to do when you're overseas, but I presume they won't airlift you a vacuum-packed meal to a beach in Bali.

Eating out and going on holiday are pleasures of life. We mustn't ignore them, or expect to manage our weight in the long term without addressing them.

A saintly, no-fun approach to weight loss is classic short-termism. It exemplifies all that's wrong with the "diet" as a way of losing weight.

If you stop eating out until you reach your desired weight, it means that you'll be ill-prepared for normal life. When your diet stops and you start eating normally, you'll gain weight. This is how yo-yo dieting happens.

What is the solution to this? You need to have ways of dealing with common situations that occur in your life, including eating out and travel.

There are many aspects of a meal eaten out of the house that lend themselves to making people eat more. These include:

1. Eating in company
2. Greater variety of foods

3. Different, novel foods
4. Feeling more relaxed

But the biggest issue as far as I can see is that we all have unconscious beliefs and assumptions that drive our behaviour. Often, we think something is true when it's not. And because of these incorrect assumptions, our actions may not be based on reality.

And we certainly have many assumptions related to eating out. Let's look at some of these in more depth, so you'll see that much of the "danger" of eating out relates back to these false assumptions.

1. Eating out is all about the food

Why do you eat out? Is it purely for the food?

Do you eat at an Italian restaurant for the food? Yes? But if it was only about the food, there'd be little difference between dinner at a nice restaurant and getting a takeaway and eating at home. No, there's more to eating out than just the food.

Eating out is about the outing itself. It's about leaving the house. It's about going somewhere different. This element of enjoying going out isn't related to how much or even what you eat. It's a pleasure in and of itself.

Similarly, when you go to a new restaurant, you derive enjoyment from the new surroundings.

It may be the decor. It may be the pleasure of being in an environment where other people are relaxed and enjoying themselves. If you go to a restaurant with company, then there's the enjoyment from socialising too.

And let's not forget the joys of having someone else cook for you and serve you the food.

Of course, none of the things I've just mentioned have anything to do with what you eat or how much you eat. And this is an important distinction.

If you think that your pleasure from eating out comes purely from how much you eat then you'll act completely differently from someone who realises that there are many enjoyable aspects of eating out, only one of which is how much you eat.

2. For me to enjoy the meal as much as possible, I need to eat as much as I can manage
This is a common belief, perhaps more so with men than women. But of course when we consider it in more detail, it's not true.

Is stuffing yourself really the path to enjoyment? Think back to a meal when you ate too much. Was feeling bloated really the way to feel pleasure?

How about a meal where you stopped earlier and felt comfortably satisfied? Realise that eating too much actually detracts from the enjoyment of the meal.

3. For me to enjoy eating out, I need to try as many different dishes as possible

This is a belief that plays itself out when people order collectively and then share dishes, or if the meal is buffet style. So if there are ten plates on offer, this belief dictates that you've extracted the most out of your dining experience if you've sampled all ten plates.

Something in us makes us feel that we're getting maximum value and enjoyment by trying everything. It's as if we're losing out if we don't sample all of the variety on offer.

As I ask my clients, if you sampled all ten dishes, what's the likelihood that you'd have enjoyed every dish you tried? Most unlikely.

There would probably be three to four dishes that you really enjoyed (if that). The rest would be either mediocre or not to your liking. And you were just forcing them down to ensure that you sampled everything.

Of course it's nice to try different foods, but when it leads to you spending most of the night having foods you don't like, then it's no longer helpful.

4. If I have to limit myself when I'm eating out, then a part of me dies inside

A melodramatic statement to be sure, but actually also a quote from one of my clients. It's a sentiment shared by many of my clients who call themselves "foodies" *(foodie n. A person who is very keen on food; a gourmet)*.

The interesting thing is that we all have to, and do, limit ourselves when we're dining out. Even the foodies.

For example, when you got to a restaurant, do you order EVERYTHING on the menu? No, of course you don't. So, in effect, you make choices. You decide which items you want and which you don't.

We all limit our intake in some ways. And so what's the difference if you limit yourself to 5 per cent of the menu or 4 per cent? It's not the end of the world and it's not the end of foodie-ness either.

I had a client who went on a wine-tasting trip. She was keen to try as many of the local wines as possible.

But when she thought about this some more, she realised that she would probably not be able to drink all the different varieties of wine in that region. So she would *always* have to limit herself.

She realised that this obsession with trying as many as possible was undermining her desire to lose weight, and she was putting unnecessary pressure on herself.

5. This is my only opportunity to eat this particular dish
Unless it literally is your last night on this planet (in which case, go for it), you'll generally have an opportunity to eat a particular food again. And if not, is eating more of this food now going to make any difference tomorrow?

Your new eating out commandments:

1. I appreciate and enjoy the non-eating aspects of eating out.
2. I only eat what I truly love and can enjoy.
3. I realise that stuffing myself doesn't mean I enjoy the meal more; in fact, it often diminishes enjoyment.

4. I don't need to try every dish in order to enjoy the meal.

Some general eating out tips:

- Raise the bar on the kind of food you eat. Don't settle for mediocre. Only eat food that's amazing. Become a connoisseur with very high standards.
- Always ask for dressing on the side.
- Load up on water, salad and soup. As chefs say, the cheapest ingredients for food are water and air.

    And for someone wanting to maximise their enjoyment and feel full with fewer calories, having a starter of soup or salad or drinking water ahead of eating is a great way to feel full sooner.
- Stick to two courses – this is a rule that I generally suggest to my clients, and most take it on board. If you go to a restaurant, pick two courses and stick to it. Make sure that you'll enjoy them. This doesn't seem like a big deal, but in the long run it can make a huge difference.

So either pick starter and main, or main and dessert. I haven't seen many clients choose starter and dessert, but that's also possible.

If you make the starter a salad or a soup, you're allowed three courses, but make sure you're eating the third course because you're hungry, not just because you want three courses.

Other scenarios

Desserts
One client of mine goes out for dinner with her husband every Sunday night. Previously, after every meal she would have a dessert, which was usually ice cream based. Harmless and understandable? As it turns out, no.

After working with me, she realised that she only really got enjoyment out of the first one to two bites. After that, she was only eating it because of the completion compulsion (see Chapter 9).

What this meant was that she was possibly consuming 300 extra calories (depending on the dessert) each time, unnecessarily. This could add up to three to four pounds over a year. It wasn't so harmless after all.

So think about this the next time you have dessert. Are you getting equal enjoyment from every bite? It's very unlikely.

So what did my dessert-eating client do? She started sharing her desserts with her husband. She would take a couple of mouthfuls to get the "hit" and then leave the rest to her husband. And when she went out with others, she shared with whoever was willing to share.

The great thing about this is that you can maximise your enjoyment without consuming extra, unnecessary calories.

Eating in a group
Eating in a group can make people eat more. In fact, the larger the group, the more food people eat.[1] People sharing a meal with one other person eat roughly 33 per cent more food.

And as the number of people at the table rises, so too does the amount of food eaten. Sharing a meal with seven other people can lead to people eating double what they'd normally eat if they were dining alone.[2]

What's also clear is that how much you eat is determined by whom you're eating with. People usually eat more when family and friends are present, but less when eating with co-workers. Women are more likely to eat more when eating with a man, but not when with a woman.[2]

And if the person you're dining with eats more, then you'll eat more.[3] We use others as a yardstick for what is an appropriate amount to eat. So eating with slim people who eat very little is a better bet than hanging out with big eaters.

Here are some strategies to overcome the challenges of eating in a group:

- Try to be the last person to start eating, and then go deliberately slowly. Try not to finish before anyone else at the table.
- Relish every bite you take.
- Benchmark yourself against the other people eating. Slow down your eating, and as a kind of game try to make sure you finish after them.
- If you know who it is, sit next to the slowest eater and pace yourself with them. I had one client who had to jostle and push people aside in order to secure her seat next to the slow eater. This isn't always necessary but I commended her keenness.
- Sit next to women rather than men at a dinner table.
- Talk a lot. The more time your mouth is talking, the less time it can be eating.
- Leave food on your plate to avoid other people shovelling more food on your plate. This applies equally to alcohol; leave your glass full to avoid top-ups.

Canapés

They are the scourge of the sociable, modern dieter. A large proportion of my clients regularly attend social and business functions and have to contend with canapés as an ever-present hazard.

Little sausages wrapped in bacon. Chicken skewers. Crostini with salmon. Delicious but dangerous.

As with any food or drink item where it's difficult to keep track of how much you've eaten, canapés can be a real problem when you want to lose weight.

So how do you deal with canapés? I tell my clients that the key is to have a quota: pick a number you're allowed to have and stick with it.

Whenever canapés are around, you only eat the number you allow yourself. So, if that number is two, then you pick the two best canapés that you see, and have those. Then stop. Because you're allowed only two, you have to be very discerning with what you choose.

Don't waste your choice on something that's mediocre.

One of my clients has chosen zero as the number of canapés that she's allowed to have. The number you choose is up to you (I wouldn't suggest ten) but the main point is that you stick to it.

By allowing yourself a quota, you don't feel deprived and you have a way of dealing with a very common situation in a sensible, sustainable way.

Holidays
The first question I ask any client when they're going on holiday is, "Do you want to come back from holiday a lesser weight, the same weight, or a heavier weight." Very few people say heavier.

Some people are happy with being the same weight, but most want to keep losing weight, even while on holiday.

And actually one of the skills I'm proudest of is helping my clients go on holiday and have a great time but still keep losing weight.

For example, one of my clients went on a four-week trip around the Greek islands and through different strategies that we discussed she managed to have a great time and still come back four pounds lighter.

The first step, then, is to acknowledge that you don't want to be heavier when you get back than when you left. This is important because it sends a powerful message to you that you can't just hope for the best. You need to make some choices and some changes.

But don't worry, every client I've worked with who's come back from holiday having lost weight has agreed that the changes don't affect their enjoyment at all.

In fact, it makes it better, because they get the thrill of the holiday and the thrill of having lost weight too. The icing on the cake.

Holiday strategies:

1. A good question that I get clients to ask themselves throughout their holiday is: Will NOT eating this particular food ruin my holiday or affect my overall enjoyment of the holiday?

   In other words, does the overall enjoyment of the holiday hinge on that one piece of food? Almost always the answer is no. The message here is that reducing what you eat won't ruin your holiday.

2. Another question to ask: Does trying every type of food in this area make it a better holiday? Is it even possible?

3. You can also ask: Will not eating this now matter much to me in 20 minutes?

4. As with canapés, have a quota for certain foods that you enjoy and so make sure when you have them that they're worth it. Again, relish every bite.
5. As I covered in Chapter 7: Balanced Indulgence, plan your meals. If you know you're going to have a big dinner, go easy on lunch.
6. Eat as much as you need to feel satisfied, and not more than that.
7. As discussed earlier, raise the bar. Only eat the best. Don't settle for food that you don't like unless it's unequivocally healthy for you.

Chapter 14 Summary

1. Question your beliefs about what constitutes a good night out.
2. Don't associate eating a lot and trying everything in the restaurant with enjoyment. They're not related.
3. You can get maximum enjoyment from desserts without excess calories.
4. Have a quality quota for canapés.
5. Use holiday strategies to come back lighter after your big break.

15

"CHOCOLATE IS CALLING": HOW TO RESIST FOOD TEMPTATION

We're surrounded by any number of temptations on a daily basis, from the chocolates in the supermarket aisle to the dessert menu at the restaurant to the bag of sweets your child is eating.

And it's a fact of life that the foods with the highest fat and sugar are often the most alluring or tasty.

We are, in fact, hard-wired to seek out and enjoy such foods because our ancestors were never sure when their next meal was going to arrive, so they had to "stock up" as much as possible. The best way to stock up is, of course, to eat high-fat, high-sugar foods.

This makes it hard to resist when treats are put in front of you.

However, if you want to reap the rewards of weight loss (improved health, energy and confidence) then how you cope with these key moments determines your success.

The mistake many would-be dieters make about temptation is that they write off slip-ups as inconsequential or inevitable.

"This won't matter, it's just one", "I've had a hard day, so I deserve this", and "The diet starts tomorrow" are all rationalisations, ways of justifying the yielding to temptation. But unfortunately, they're also all fantasy.

It's like the old joke that taking food from someone else's plate doesn't count as calories. Let's not kid ourselves: everything we eat contains calories.

We can justify it all we like, but if you recall the example from earlier, one can of coke per day can add up to ten to fourteen pounds of weight in a year. So even the smallest amounts count. Why waste your calorie allowance on something you hadn't intended to eat anyway?

Some people feel that the only way to respond to temptation is willpower. They think they must maintain rigid self-discipline for the rest of their lives.

No wonder so many people feel terrified about losing weight. What a depressing thought! Fortunately, there are more reliable and easier ways to resist temptation.

Control your environment
It's easier to control your environment than rely on will-power. Another way to look at it is that the best way to resist temptation is to avoid it.

This sounds obvious, but most people aren't very good at this. Instead, their environment is set up so that they're continually being tempted.

If someone places a box of chocolates near your desk at work, move them further away. Preferably out of your line of sight. Simply having treats in your line of sight makes it more likely that you'll eat them.

Similarly, if a particular route you take while walking or in the car takes you past somewhere where you know you'll be tempted, then go a different way.

For instance, if you know it's going to be too hard to walk past that cake shop without popping in then don't walk past. Seems simple enough, but most people don't even think about it.

Also, if you find it hard to resist when you have treats at home then don't keep them at home. If you have to, for the kids, then keep them in a cupboard that's separate from the rest of your food at home so that you don't have to keep looking at them every time you go into the kitchen.

If a treat is near you or in front of you, you'll have an argument in your mind about whether to eat it or not, and every so often you'll lose the argument.

This alone can mean many extra calories per day and consequently many extra pounds on your waistline. If the food isn't there, there's no argument.

Look at your daily routine and see whether you can reduce your exposure to foods that you like eating but know that they hinder you in getting to your weight goal.

How much of your day is spent resisting temptation?
Realise that while temptation is all around you, only a few moments a day are danger times. Think about it. In a 24-hour period, how much time do you spend resisting temptation? If it's more than a few minutes then you're not controlling your environment well enough (see the earlier section).

These feelings of temptation aren't permanent.

When you're faced with a chocolate cake dessert after dinner, does the temptation last for the next 24 hours? Do you spend every waking moment thinking what it would have been like to eat it? Do you wake up in the middle of the night in a cold sweat regretting your decision?

In actuality the temptation lasts a few seconds, or a few minutes at most. And if resisted, it's followed by relief, not regret.

And so the decision you have to make is, do I tolerate the few seconds of temptation to then enjoy my new weight, or do I give in to the temptation and then spend many hours or more trying to lose the weight? As they say, "a minute on the lips, a lifetime on the hips".

Ask the right questions
How you deal with tempting food often comes down to the questions that you ask yourself right before you make the decision to have or not have it.

As an example, imagine that you're eating out at a restaurant.

You've had the main meal, and the waiter has brought you the dessert menu. When you look at the menu a particular dessert catches your eye.

Even though you're seeing me tomorrow at my clinic for another weight loss session, you're very tempted. At this point, most people would ask themselves

"Do I have the dessert or not?"

This seems like a reasonable question to ask. But actually, by asking yourself this particular question you've made it very hard to resist the dessert. When you ask yourself, "Do I have the dessert or not?" you're giving yourself a very loaded choice.

The choice is between having something sweet and indulgent that you'd probably enjoy the taste of OR depriving yourself of that enjoyable experience.

In other words, do you let yourself have something enjoyable or not? Of course, it's natural to choose the enjoyable option. So is it any wonder that most people, when faced with the temptation of dessert, can't resist?

However, in reality, the choice you're faced with is NOT whether to have dessert or not, it's whether you want to **lose weight or not**. Remember, every mouthful of food you have has an impact on your weight.

So the question you should instead be asking yourself is:

> *"Do I want to lose weight or not?"* or even
> *"Do I want to slow down my progress in losing weight?"* or
> *"Do I want this, even though I know the feeling will pass and I'll feel guilty afterwards?"*

You need to keep clear in your mind your reasons for wanting to lose weight. Do you want to feel healthier? Do you want to fit into new clothes? Do you want to feel more energetic, more attractive and better about yourself?

If you're clear on your reasons for losing weight and you see the dessert as something that may prevent you from achieving those goals then you'll be making your decision about whether or not to have the dessert with much more awareness.

Get in the habit of asking the right questions when faced with tempting food. You may still choose to eat it (and that's okay) but always do so with full awareness. And if you choose to eat it, make sure you enjoy every mouthful and stop when it's no longer enjoyable.

Delay, don't deny
Another very effective strategy that a lot of my clients seem to really find useful is the idea of delaying instead of denying.

When faced with the temptation to have a treat, wait 20 minutes before deciding to have it. This 20-minute delay is almost like your test for whether you really want the treat or whether it's just a passing whim.

In most cases, especially at the end of a meal, if you wait 20 minutes, you'll find that you're no longer hungry and no longer desire the treat.

What this means is that instead of denying yourself something (which to your mind feels like deprivation) you're simply delaying when you eat it. This might seem like semantics but it makes a huge difference to your coping abilities. We hate denial, but most of us can tolerate delay.

Have a "quality quota"
I often use the quality quota (as mentioned in Chapter 14: Having a Life) with my weight loss clients, especially in the holiday periods.

For instance, if a client especially likes Christmas puddings, she's allowed to set a quota, an amount that she's allowed to have over the Christmas period. Let's say that number is three. Of course, what quota you set is up to you (taking into account your weight goals and desire to achieve them as soon as possible!).

With the quota, let's say this client can have up to three Christmas puddings over the whole Christmas period (from 12th December to 3rd January).

But the caveat is that if she has a Christmas pudding, she must make sure that it is the FINEST, HIGHEST-QUALITY Christmas pudding that she can find.

She isn't to settle for substandard pudding. To paraphrase one of my clients, "If I'm going to have the calories, I might as well make sure they're the best."

The quality quota means that you never have to deprive yourself again. You know that you're allowed to eat whatever you want. All you have to do is choose *when* you have it. It also ensures that you raise the bar of quality of the food that you eat.

Chapter 15 Summary

1. Temptation is all around but you can use other ways that work better than willpower to fight it.
2. Controlling your environment is much easier than using willpower.
3. Ask the right questions. Every decision has a consequence, so bring to the forefront the real impact of eating something.

4. Temptation only lasts a few key moments. Master those and you master your temptation.
5. Delay don't deny.
6. Use a quality quota to enjoy what you want but not overdo it.

16

STAYING SLIM: HOW TO MAINTAIN YOUR WEIGHT LOSS

There are many ways to lose weight. Some are healthy, others are not. But there's only one way to maintain weight loss and that's by changing your habits.

There's only one way to maintain your weight.

That has been the principle behind this entire book: safe, effective weight loss that lasts.

What's the alternative? Of course, it's going on a diet, losing some weight and then as soon as you come off the diet, gaining the weight back again. The yo-yo diet phenomenon.

If you're overweight, it can be tempting to ignore the whole concept of maintenance of weight. After all, most people are totally focused on how to lose weight. It seems like putting the cart before the horse to worry about what to do after you've lost weight.

But this is short-sighted and pretty much the problem with most fad diets. They focus exclusively on how to lose weight and pay no attention to the fact that you need to live with your new weight for the rest of your life.

As I've mentioned throughout this book, you want to begin in the way that you intend to continue. Unrealistic, drastic changes aren't sustainable, so I don't use them. I want my clients to make easy changes that they know they can maintain forever.

And as I stated in Chapter 10: Exercise, don't do anything that you don't think you can maintain for the rest of your life. And always be thinking of the future. Is this sustainable?

Once you've reached your goal weight, you must pay attention to maintenance, because if you don't you'll start gaining weight again.

One of the big challenges that my clients face is that maintaining weight isn't as exciting as losing weight.

When we're in weight loss phase, there's an almost game-like quality to the process. There are victories almost every week, with developing new behaviours, seeing the weight fall on the scales and noticing that clothes fit better.

Once the weight has been lost, however, there's less positive feedback and fewer new victories. So you need to sustain your interest and commitment to staying thin.

But as well as that, I think the key to maintenance is having a plan. Instead of leaving things to chance, you need to prepare for how you're going to live your life as a slim person.

The first thing that you need to focus on is daily weighing.

This is very important. Regular monitoring of your weight is far better than one day realising that your jeans no longer fit, which is the usual way people realise that they've gained weight. And by then it may be too late, or at least much more difficult to get things back to where they were.

Once you've reached your goal weight, instead of trying to stick to that particular weight, it's much easier and more useful to have a weight range. The range allows for the normal fluctuations in weight that I've already talked about.

A good way to think of this is tramlines.[2] This is an upper and lower weight that you're comfortable with. Your aim is to stay within the tramlines. When the weight strays either above or below the tramlines then you know you have to do something about it.

In addition to having tramlines, you need to establish a procedure that kicks in as soon as you stray off track. The procedure is up to you to establish, but don't wait till after you've left the tramlines to establish it!

This is what I suggest for my clients if they go above the tramline (upper weight limit):

1. Restart the food diary.
2. Contact me immediately.
3. Review reasons why you wanted to manage your weight at this level.
4. Remember that you have the tools necessary to regain control of your weight.

What we're aiming to do is get control over your routine as quickly as possible. Your weight may have strayed above the tramline because you lost awareness of what you were eating, or just got complacent.

By starting the food diary you introduce immediate awareness. Contacting me enables my clients to get an objective viewpoint and advice for regaining momentum.

I get clients to review the reasons that they wanted to manage their weight, because it can be so easy to forget what things were like when they were overweight.

All the negatives of being overweight can easily be overlooked and therefore the significance of regaining weight can be ignored. This is dangerous.

If you let things slip too far, it makes it much harder to get back under control.

Better to respond quickly when it's easier than wait too long. Part of this is reminding yourself of all the benefits of being slim and the negatives of being overweight.

It's also important to remember that if you've followed the advice in this book and applied it in order to lose weight then you have all the tools and strategies you need to get back on track.

That is a real feather in your cap and it's more than most people have. It puts you in an enviable position.

You're far better placed to get back to your ideal weight than others in a similar situation.

The fourth strategy for weight loss maintenance is regular exercise.

As we saw in the chapter on exercise, physical activity isn't helpful on its own for weight loss, but studies have shown that it's one of the most consistent factors in people who maintain weight loss.[3,4]

Is that to say that you can't maintain weight without exercise? No. It's possible to stay at a certain weight without exercise. But exercise makes it easier.

One of the reasons why is possibly that someone who's motivated enough to maintain exercise will be more likely to stick with an eating pattern that maintains their weight. And of course with all the other positive benefits of exercise, why wouldn't you?

Again, as I mentioned in Chapter 10 on exercise, choose ways of increasing activity that you're likely to stick to. Use anticipated regret to make sure you stick to the habit. And always remember that lifestyle activity is as effective for managing your weight as formal, structured exercise.

The final part of the maintenance plan should be anticipating high-risk situations.

For each of us there may be an infinite number of situations that could happen to derail our weight management, but in reality, most of us could identify a few situations that are more likely than others.

Here are a few that clients have identified in the past:

1. Going on holiday
2. Change of circumstance; for example spending large amounts of time at home
3. Socialising
4. Crisis (this can be things like job loss, relationship break-up, loss of a loved one or health problems).

Anything that leads to you losing focus can result in weight gain. This is especially true of crises, where your attention is diverted to other matters and paying attention to your weight seems less important.

Of course, neglecting your weight can have implications on your health that can make problems even worse. One of the keys to maintaining weight loss is to catch small slip-ups and ensure that they don't turn into bigger weight gains.[5]

The next section is about how to manage the mental game of weight management, which is crucial in times of crisis.

The mental game of weight loss

A large part of maintaining your weight comes down to psychology. Let's review some of the key concepts of maintaining weight.

Of course, much of this depends on you maintaining your focus and motivation to lose weight. Indeed, in many ways, the only time your weight maintenance can go wrong is if you take your eye off the ball.

In other words, if things go wrong, you must be motivated enough to do something about it, rather than saying, "Oh well, I'll deal with it later."

First of all, your biggest enemy is complacency. This is when you start to believe that maintaining weight is too easy and you stop doing the right things.

Remember, even once you've learned how to eat what you want and still manage your weight, you're not superhuman. If you eat too much, you'll still gain weight. This applies to everyone.

Weight maintenance *is* easy, but you still need to keep doing what got you there.

The other big danger is forgetting the benefits of losing weight.

Some people may notice their weight increase over the upper tramline and not be motivated to do anything about it. This arises from thinking that the inconvenience of maintaining is more troublesome than the pain of being overweight.

This can easily happen if you forget what things were like when you were overweight. And believe me, this is easy to do. I'm constantly reminding my clients of how much has changed since they were overweight to ensure they never forget and keep motivated to stay on the path.

Acknowledge all the things that are possible now that you're slimmer, compared to when you were overweight: things like fitting into slimmer, stylish clothes, and feeling more energetic and confident. All of these things should be powerful motivators to keep up the good work.

As I say to my clients, now that you've lost the weight, the stakes are much higher. Knowing the mental effort it took to get here, and knowing how bad things were when you were overweight, would you really want to jeopardise it?

As I've said earlier, every decision about eating is not "Should I eat it or not?" but "Should I jeopardise my progress or not?".

These things may be hard to do when you're in a crisis, but that's all the more reason to plan some kind of response ahead of time.

It may be tempting to just ignore it and comfort-eat, but the anticipation of these problems ahead of time will make you better prepared.

Reframe the work needed; it's worth it
I had a client who had lost two stone (28 pounds) and was thinking about maintenance. She said it would be awfully sad (as in pitiful) if she had to keep on recording a food diary.

But as I pointed out, if 80 seconds filling out a food diary was all that stood between maintaining her new weight and sliding back into ill-fitting jeans, feeling self-conscious and lacking energy, then it was a very, very small price to pay.

Think of the effort of starting another diet again. It's not worth it.

Is it hard to maintain your weight?
The good news is that the longer you maintain your weight, the easier it gets. The evidence is that people who maintain their weight loss for more than two years have a 50 per cent less chance of weight regain.[6] And as people lose weight, the effort they need to put in reduces.[7]

This would tie in with habit formation being ingrained into your mind so that it becomes second nature. This will, of course, vary between people, but once the habits become something you no longer need to think about, you have a much better chance of maintaining your weight.

The fact that the strategies you have learned in this book focus directly on changing your habits will make this process even more effective.

Lastly, one of the factors associated with successful weight maintenance is maintaining regular contact with someone who can keep you accountable.[8,9,10]

Do you think that after losing weight your chances of success in maintaining your weight would be increased by having someone check in with you and make sure that you were still on track? Yes. Having someone to review your progress makes a big difference in a person's ability to maintain their weight loss.

And that's why I ensure that I maintain regular contact with my clients even after they've achieved their weight loss goals. This means that I catch up with them at least every six months.

During these appointments the main priority is to ensure that they haven't drifted from the original behaviours that were the reason for their success in the first place.

Ask yourself who could support you even after you've lost weight. This could be a personal trainer or a nutritionist.

Even if the person isn't directly familiar with this particular programme, the benefit lies simply with having someone to keep you accountable for the long term. You should ideally see them regularly (at least every six months).

Chapter 16 Summary

1. Maintenance is what most diets ignore, yet it's the only way to avoid yo-yo dieting.
2. When you follow the principles of this book, you're much better placed to maintain your weight loss.
3. Having a plan is crucial.
4. Weigh yourself regularly and have a weight range that you want to stick to (marked out by tramlines – an upper and lower weight limit).
5. Have a plan in place in case you stray outside your desired weight range.
6. Exercise regularly.
7. Anticipate high-risk situations.
8. Handle the mental game of weight maintenance, especially complacency.
9. Get support for the long term.

EXTRAS TO HELP YOU GET SLIM AND HEALTHY WITHOUT DIETING

One way to learn more about the principles discussed in this book is to visit my website:

www.DoctorKWeightLoss.com

Here you can find:

- more weight loss tips.
- articles.
- online courses that take you step-by-step through losing weight without dieting.

And if you really want to make sure you lose weight once and for all, you can find information on the site about getting my personal help to lose weight at my clinic in London.

NOTES

Chapter 1

1. Muraven, M and Baumeister, RF (2000). Self-regulation and depletion of limited resources: Does self-control resemble a muscle? *Psychological Bulletin*, 126:247–259.
2. Muraven, M, Tice, DM, and Baumeister RF (1998). Self-control as a limited resource: Regulatory depletion patterns. *Journal of Personality and Social Psychology*, 74:774–789.

Chapter 3

1. Wing, R and Phelan, S (2005). Long-term weight loss maintenance. *American Journal of Clinical Nutrition*, 82(suppl):222S–5S.
2. Ibid
3. Blackburn, G (1995). Effect of degree of weight loss on health benefits. Obesity Research, 3: 211S–216S.

Chapter 4

1. Schweitzer, D., Dubois, E., Doel-Tanis, N., and Oei, H. (2007). Successful weight loss surgery

improved eating control and energy metabolism: A review of the evidence. *Obesity Surgery*, 17: 533–539.
2. Kausman, R. (1998) *If Not Dieting, Then What?* NSW: Griffin.

Chapter 5

1. Havel, PJ (2001). Peripheral signals conveying metabolic information to the brain: short-term and long-term regulation of food intake and energy homeostasis. *Experimental Biology and Medicine* (Maywood), 226: 963–77.
2. Macias, AE (2004). Experimental demonstration of human weight homeostasis: implications for understanding obesity. *British Journal of Nutrition*, 91: 479–484.

Chapter 6

1. Wadden, TA, Berkowitz, RI, Womble, LG, Sarwer, DB, Phelan, S, Cato, RK, Hesson, LA, Osei, SY, Kaplan, R, and Stunkard, AJ (2005). Randomized trial of lifestyle modification and pharmacotherapy for obesity. New England Journal of Medicine, 353:2111–2120.

2. Baker, RC and Kirschenbaum, DS (1993). Self-monitoring may be necessary for successful weight control. *Behavior Therapy*, 24: 377–394.
3. Schnoll, R and Zimmerman, BJ (2001). Self-regulation training enhances dietary self-efficacy and dietary fiber consumption. *Journal of the American Dietetic Association*, 101: 1006–1011.
4. Livingstone, MB and Black, AE (2003). Markers of the validity of reported energy intake. *Journal of Nutrition*, 133(suppl): 895S–920S.
5. Lichtman, SW, Pisarska, K, Berman, ER, Pestone, M, Dowling, H, Offenbacher, E, Weisel, H, Heshka, S, Matthews, DE, and Heymsfield, SB (1992). Discrepancy between self-reported and actual caloric intake and exercise in obese subjects. *New England Journal of Medicine*, 327: 1893–1898.
6. Mertz, W, Tsui, JC, Judd, JT, Reiser, S, Hallfrisch, J, Morris, ER, Steele, PD, and Lashley, E (1991). What are people really eating? The relation between energy intake derived from estimated diet records and intake determined to maintain body weight. *American Journal of Clinical Nutrition*, 54: 291–295.
7. Racette, SB, Weiss, EP, Schechtman, KB, Steger-May, K, Villareal, DT, Obert, KA, and Holloszy,

JO (2008). Influence of weekend lifestyle patterns on body weight. *Obesity* (Silver Spring), 16(8): 1826–1830.

Chapter 7

1. Mattes, RD, Pierce, CB, and Friedman, MI (1988). Daily caloric intake of normal-weight adults: Response to changes in dietary energy density of a luncheon meal. *American Journal of Clinical Nutrition*, 48: 214–219.
2. Ebbeling, CB, Sinclair, KB, Pereira, MA, Garcia-Lago, E, Feldman, HA, and Ludwig, DS (2004). Compensation for energy intake from fast food among overweight and lean adolescents. *JAMA*, 2004, 291: 2828–2833.
3. U.S. Department of Health and Human Services, U.S. Department of Agriculture (2005). *Dietary Guidelines for Americans 2005*. Washington (DC): Government Printing Office.

Chapter 8

1. Andrade, AM, Greene, GW, and Melanson, KJ (2008). Eating slowly led to decreases in energy intake within meals in healthy women, *Journal of the American Dietetic Association*, 108: 1186–1191.

2. Sasaki, S, Katagiri, A, Tsuji, T, Shimoda, T, and Amano, K (2003). Self-reported rate of eating correlates with body mass index in 18-year-old Japanese women, *International Journal of Obesity*, 27: 1405–1410.

3. Maruyama, K, Sato, S, Ohira, T, Maeda, K, Noda, H, Kubota, Y, Nishimura, S, Kitamura, A, Kiyama, M, Okada, T, Imano, H, Nakamura, M, Ishikawa, Y, Kurokawa, M, Sasaki, S, Iso, H (2008). The joint impact on being overweight of self reported behaviours of eating quickly and eating until full: cross sectional survey, *British Medical Journal*, 337: a2002.

4. Laessle, RG, Lehrke, S, and Duckers, S (2007). Laboratory eating behavior in obesity. *Appetite*, 49: 399–404.

5. Viskaal-van Dongen, M, Kok, FJ, and de Graaf, C (2011). Eating rate of commonly consumed foods promotes food and energy intake. *Appetite*, 56: 25–31.

6. Andrade, AM, Greene, GW, and Melanson, KJ (2008). Eating slowly led to decreases in energy intake within meals in healthy women, *Journal of the American Dietetic Association*, 108: 1186–1191.

7. Spiegel, TA, Wadden, TA, Foster, GD. (1991) Objective measurement of eating rate during behavioral treatment of obesity, *Behavior Therapy*, 22: 61–67.

8. Paintal, AS (1954). A study of gastric stretch receptors. Their role in the peripheral mechanism of satiation of hunger and thirst. *The Journal of Physiology*, 126: 255–270.

9. Murphy, KG and Bloom, SR (2004). Gut hormones in the control of appetite. *Experimental Physiology*, 89: 507–516.

10. Kokkinos, A, Le Roux, CW, Alexiadou, K, Tentolouris, N, Vincent, RP, Kyriaki, D, *et al.* (2009). Eating slowly increases the postprandial response of the anorexigenic gut hormones, peptide YY and glucagon-like eptide-1. *Journal of Clinical Endocrinology and Metabolism*, 95: 333–337.

11. Zijlstra, N, de Wijk, RA, Mars, M, Stafleu, A and de Graaf, C (2009). Effect of bite size and oral processing time of a semisolid food on satiation. *American Journal of Clinical Nutrition*, 90: 269–275.

Chapter 9

1. Rolls, BJ, Roe, LS, Kral, TV, Meengs, JS, and Wall, DE (2004). Increasing the portion size of a packaged snack increases energy intake in men and women. *Appetite*, 42: 63–69.

2. Rolls, BJ, Morris, EL, and Roe, LS (2002). Portion size of food affects energy intake in normal-weight

and overweight men and women. *American Journal of Clinical Nutrition*, 76: 1207–1213.

3. Geier, AB, Rozin, P, and Doros, G (2006). Unit bias. A new heuristic that helps explain the effect of portion size on food intake. *Psychological Science*, 17(6): 521–525.

4. Siegel, PS (1957). The completion compulsion in human eating. *Psychological Reports*, 3: 15–16.

5. Wansink, B, Painter, JE, and North, J (2005). Bottomless bowls: Why visual cues of portion size may influence food intake. *Obesity Research*, 13: 93–100.

6. Wansink, B, Van Ittersum, K, and Painter, JE (2006). Ice cream illusions: Bowl size, spoon size, and serving size. *American Journal of Preventive Medicine*, 31(3): 240–243.

Chapter 10

1. Donnelly, JE, Hill, JO, Jacobsen, DJ, Potteiger, J, Sullivan, DK, Johnson, SL, Heelan, K, Hise, M, Fennessey, PV, Sonko, B, Sharp, T, Jakicic, JM, Blair, SN, Tran, ZV, Mayo, M, Gibson, C, and Washburn, RA (2003). Effects of a 16-month randomized controlled exercise trial on body weight and composition in young, overweight men and women: The Midwest Exercise Trial. *Archives of Internal Medicine*, 163: 1343–1350.

2. Nieman, DC, Brock, DW, Butterworth, D, Utter, AC, and Nieman, CW (2002). Reducing diet and/or exercise training decreases the lipid and lipoprotein risk factors of moderately obese women. *Journal of the American College of Nutrition*, 21: 344–350.

3. Hinkleman, LL and Nieman, DC (1993). The effects of a walking program on body composition and serum lipids and lipoproteins in overweight women. *Journal of Sports Medicine and Physical Fitness*, 33: 49–58.

4. Pate, RR, Pratt, M, Blair, SN, Haskell, WL, Macera, CA, Bouchard, C, Buchner, D, Ettinger, W, Heath, GW, King, AC, Kriska, A, Leon, AS, Marcus, BH, Morris, J, Paffenbarger, RS, Patrick, K, Pollock, ML, Rippe, JM, Sallis, J, and Wilmore, JH (1995). Physical activity and public health: a recommendation from the Centers for Disease Control and Prevention and the American College of Sports Medicine. *Journal of the American Medical Association*, 273: 402–407.

5. Miller, WC, Koceja, DM, and Hamilton, EJ (1997). A meta-analysis of the past 25 years of weight loss research using diet, exercise or diet plus exercise intervention. *International Journal of Obesity and Related Metabolic Disorders*, 21: 941–947.

6. Klem, ML, Wing, RR, McGuire, MT, Seagle, HM, and Hill, JO (1997). A descriptive study of individuals successful at long-term maintenance of substantial weight loss. *American Journal of Clinical Nutrition*, 66: 239–246.

7. The NHS Information Centre, Lifestyles Statistics (10 February 2010). Statistics on obesity, physical activity and diet: England, 2010. Online at http://www.ic.nhs.uk/pubs/opad10 (accessed June 2011).

8. Abraham, C and Sheeran, P (2004). Deciding to exercise: The role of anticipated regret. *British Journal of Health Psychology*, 9: 269–278.

9. Anderson, RE, Wadden, TA, Bartlett, SJ, Zemel, B, Verde, TJ, and Franckowiak, SC (1999). Effects of lifestyle activity vs structured aerobic exercise in obese women. *Journal of the American Medical Association*, 281: 335–340.

10. Andersen, RE, Franckowiak, SC, Bartless, SJ, and Fontaine, KR (2002). Physiologic changes after diet combined with structured aerobic exercise or lifestyle activity. *Metabolism*, 51: 1528–1533.

11. Dunn, AL, Marcus, BH, Kampert, JB, Garcia, ME, Kohl, HW, and Blair, SN (1999). Comparison of lifestyle and structured interventions to increase physical activity and cardiorespiratory fitness. *Journal of the American Medical Association* 281: 327–334.

12. Jakicic, JM, Wing, RR, Butler, BA, and Robertson, RJ (1995). Prescribing exercise in multiple short bouts versus one continuous bout: effects on adherence, cardiorespiratory fitness, and weight loss in over-weight women. *International Journal of Obesity*, 19: 893–901.

13. DeBusk, RF, Stenestrand, U, Sheehan, M, and Haskell, WL (1990). Training effects of long versus short bouts of exercise in healthy subjects. *American Journal of Cardiology*, 65: 1010–1013.

Chapter 11

1. Wansink, B (2009). *Mindless Eating.* London: Hay House.

2. Wansink, B, Painter, JE, and Lee, YK (2006). The office candy dish: Proximities influence on estimated and actual consumption. *International Journal of Obesity*, 30: 871–875.

Chapter 12

1. Jeffery. RW, Wing. RR, and Randall, RM (1998). Are smaller weight losses or more achievable weight loss goals better in the long term for obese patients? *Journal of Consulting and Clinical Psychology*, 66: 641–645.

Chapter 13

1. Beck, J. (2008). *The Beck Diet Solution*. London: Robinson.

Chapter 14

1. de Castro, JM, and de Castro, ES (1989). Spontaneous meal patterns in humans: Influence of the presence of other people. *American Journal of Clinical Nutrition*, 50: 23.

2. de Castro, JM (2000). Eating behavior: Lessons from the real world of humans. *Nutrition,* 16: 800–813.

3. Levitsky, DA (2005). The non-regulation of food intake in humans: Hope for reversing the epidemic of obesity. *Physiology and Behaviour,* 86: 623–632.

Chapter 16

1. Wing, RR and Phelan, S (2005). Long-term weight loss maintenance. *American Journal of Clinical Nutrition*, 82(suppl): 222S–225S.

2. Cooper, Z, Fairburn, CF, and Hawker, DM (2003). *Cognitive-behavioral Treatment of Obesity. A Clinician's Guide.* New York, NY: Guilford Press.

3. Anderson, JW, Konz, EC, Frederich, RC, and Wood, CL (2001). Long-term weight loss maintenance:

A meta-analysis of US studies. *American Journal of Clinical Nutrition*, Nov 74(5): 579–584.

4. Kayman, S, Bruvold, W, and Stern, JS (1990). Maintenance and relapse after weight loss in women: behavioral aspects. *American Journal of Clinical Nutrition*, 52: 800–807.

5. Wing, RR and Phelan, S (2005). Long-term weight loss maintenance. *American Journal of Clinical Nutrition*, 82(suppl): 222S–225S.

6. Wing, RR and Hill, JO (2001). Successful weight loss maintenance. *Annual Review of Nutrition*, 21: 323–341.

7. Klem, ML, Wing, RR, Lang, W, McGuire, MT, and Hill, JO (2000). Does weight loss maintenance become easier over time? *Obesity Research*, Sep 8(6):438–444.

8. Latner, JD, Stunkard, AJ, Wilson, GT, and Jackson, ML. The perceived effectiveness of continuing care and group support in the long-term self-help treatment of obesity. *Obesity Research*, 14: 464–471.

9. National Heart, Lung, and Blood Institute (1998). *Clinical Guidelines on the Identification, Evaluation, and Treatment of Overweight and Obesity in Adults: The Evidence Report.* Bethesda MD: National Heart, Lung, and Blood Institute.

10. Perri, MG (1998). The maintenance of treatment effects in the longterm management of obesity. *Clinical Psychology – Science and Practice*, 5: 526–543.

ABOUT THE AUTHOR

Dr Khandee Ahnaimugan is a medical doctor, author and weight loss expert, based in London, England.

His focus is on helping women over 40 to lose weight without dieting or deprivation.

Dr. Ahnaimugan's clinic is based in London's Harley Street, where clients visit him from all over the world. He has also helped thousands of women through his online weight loss programs.

For more information visit:

www.DoctorKWeightLoss.com

FURTHER READING

If you enjoyed this book, you may also enjoy:

Losing Weight After 40: How to Change Your Life Without Dieting or Deprivation

Printed in Great Britain
by Amazon